The Healing Project
How to Be Healthy and Live Well

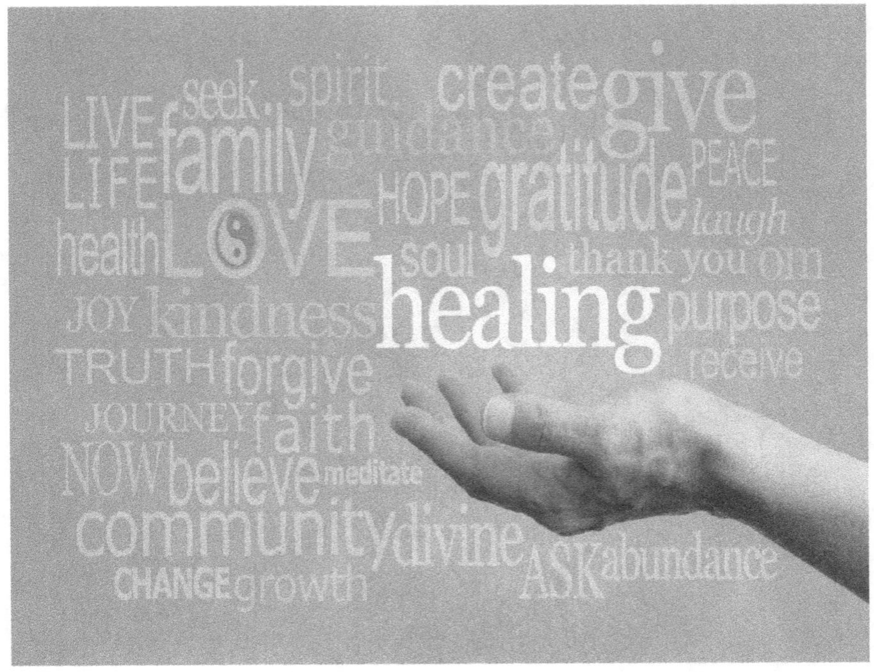

By Dr. George Samuels, M.D. (A.M.), A.M.P.

The Healing Project
How to Be Healthy and Live Well

Dedication

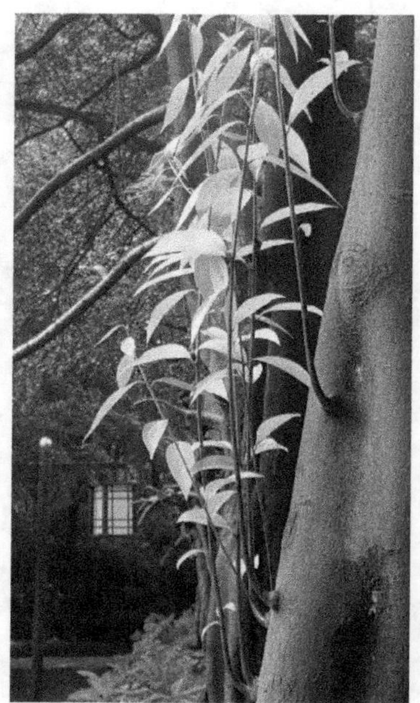

Believe
You can heal
And you can heal yourself
And Live Well!

"It is health that is real wealth and not pieces of gold and silver."
(Mahatma)
This is dedicated to my Mom who understood Holistic Health and Natural Healing

The Healing Project
How to Be Healthy and Live Well

Prologue

Join us in, becoming a part of the Healing Project and change your life, heal yourself and help us heal others and pass the word on to the entire planet.

How can we help you, and how can you help others? When is the opportunity to heal what ails you, so that you can be healed, balanced and also live well?

This project is for all and focuses on the basic ideal that we can be healthy, "wholistically," and heal whatever ails us....

... And live well!

The Healing Project
How to Be Healthy and Live Well

Introduction

Are we living well or surviving? Is this my life or your life, trying to survive another day? Have we subjected our family to a life surviving, or are we teaching them and exposing them to a life living well? Do you know the difference, or is there a difference? Is your concern only surviving? Why? Did you know you are supposed to live well, not just survive? Are you doing what it takes to survive, or live well? Only you know, but it is time we explore this and change if needed from surviving to living well. It is only our decision to just survive, or to live well.

Welcome to The Healing Project. *The sage says he will never come to heal you; why?* Reason one is the sage comes before you get sick and teaches you to be healthy, so you don't get sick. The second reason is, the sage will teach you to heal yourself. The third reason is, the sage will expect that you are doing what is vital to insure you stay healthy. Fourth, the Sage *Master* expects you to not only survive, but to live well. The primary premise is that you can heal. The secondary premise is that you can heal yourself. The third premise is that you can heal naturally utilizing alternative traditional or modern techniques. The fourth premise is that you are living well.

We are here to help you to be healthy and live well. We will, over the course of this project, provide information and insights into how to be and stay healthy. Besides surviving, some of us are experiencing non-communicable diseases that hamper our living healthy and well. We want to decrease the escalating non-communicable diseases (NCDs) that are a problem around the world. These NCDs can be reduced or eliminated when we embark on a life journey of living well, which includes activities that will help prevent non-communicable diseases. Some NCDs are heart attacks, strokes, diabetes and high blood pressure, to name a few. Some risk factors of non-communicable diseases include the environment, lifestyle or background, such as the genetics, age, and gender of a person, and exposure to air pollution. Some behaviors such as a lack of physical activity, poor diet or smoking, which could lead to obesity or hypertension, can also increase the risk of developing some non-communicable diseases. Many of these are considered preventable because the condition can be improved by removing the at-risk behavior.

Preventing NCDs requires education, information, activities and changes in our lifestyle. We can have the Doctors and medical professionals decide what is required and prescribe what is needed, but at the same time, we must take responsibility and share knowledge and information on how to heal, and how you can heal yourself. The ideal of living well is to do those things on a daily basis that improve health and the ability to live well, thereby removing or reducing at-risk behavior.

This book and project *"The Healing Project"*, will feature modules that will deal with a variety of essential categories, such as the body, mind, and spirit. This will include touchstones on general health, balance of mind, body and spirit, healing, the causes and solutions, longevity, and how to correct the imbalances in our lives through a variety of alternative and traditional ways that are non-invasive. These include such solutions as Dao yin exercises, diet, meditation, massage, qigong, Taijiquan, and specific remedies designed to heal any abnormalities. We will focus on a variety of causes and solutions tailored to support not only the individual, but also groups of people.

This *"The Healing Project"*, is a living book and a live project in, which we will create a book and a series of videos so that one can view these from their home and create a facility to answer questions and provide essential counseling and face to face consultations if at all possible. Look for our first introductory video and signups, and also to receive emails and other public media.

Have you asked yourself what it would take for you to live well? Are you living well? Do you want to live well? Are you ready for change and ready to change whatever needs to change for you to heal and begin to live well? If so, then let us begin!

The Healing Project
How to Be Healthy and Live Well

Other Titles by the Author

Audacity of Poetry,
Healing in a Word,
With Poetry in Mind,
This is Our Word,
There is Only Music Brother,
Doors to Ancient Poetical Echoes,
Lovers Should Never Quarrel,
The Song of Life,
Calm is the Water
The Healer Within Us
Mastering The Art of Taijiquan

.

The Healing Project
How to Be Healthy and Live Well

Table of Contents

I

Methodology

Again Welcome to the Healing Project

Now is the opportunity to heal what ails you, so that you can be balanced, healed and live well? The methodology of this program is to offer information, advice and services to all in need and focuses on the basic ideal that we can be healthy and heal whatever ails us so we can live well.

There are many facets to the health and wellbeing of individuals, and it requires learning and understanding that we are all whole, total beings that include our physical, mental and spiritual wellbeing. This is endowed to all of us, and we have the ability to learn and understand what this means to each and every one of us. We all have needs and requirements to have and maintain our health and wellbeing so that we can live well. We talk about living well, but many times, we don't know what that means and how to accomplish it. We go about our daily business and are busy without spending sufficient time deciding on or dissecting our movements and doings to determine if we are living well. Many say, "I am (my family is) just trying to survive!"

We assume we are ok until something happens to change our thinking. Then we determine, if there is a problem, if we should ignore or pay attention to it, or visit a health professional to assist us and determine what is going on. Since most times we are ill equipped to handle some problems, we don't pay attention to what is happening until it is an emergency situation. When the emergency happens, we then run to a doctor or hospital to fix the problem(s). Or, we swallow some pills that are marketed on TV as a general panacea, with numerous side effects that can harm some individuals more than the basic symptoms they are displaying or cause confusion with other symptoms, which may cause a person to become ill or even further out of balance. The worst is that they turn our lives into a panacea of survival.

For example, if we have one of the non-communicable diseases (NCDs) we do not know what to do when there is an emergency except go to the doctor or see a health professional. We do not think about the idea of what we should be doing to avoid these diseases, especially since many of these diseases are avoidable. We must stop the escalating non-communicable diseases that are preventable. Some of these are heart attacks, strokes, diabetes, and high blood pressure, to name a few. These are the diseases that can be eliminated when we embark on a life journey of living well, which includes activities that will help prevent non-communicable diseases. How to prevent or stop non-communicable diseases that plague us requires education, information, activities and changes in our lifestyle. As part of "The Healing Project," we will focus on how NCDs affect our living well, and we will discuss more about NCDs later on in another chapter in the book.

Our method in the healing project is to discuss health, healing and how to change our lives to live as well as we can. This works by providing details and information to increase our knowledge of what it is to live well, be in good health and heal ourselves, so as to add quality and balance or begin to change our lives in order to live well.

We will create a series of programs that will explore all facets of wellness in our complex lives to determine what each one of us needs to be balanced, in great health, healed and to live well into our future.

The methods we will employ will feature modules that focus on a variety of essential categories dealing with the body, mind, and spirit. This will include touchstones on general health, balance of mind, body and spirit, healing, the causes and solutions, longevity, and how to correct the imbalances in our lives through a variety of alternative and traditional ways.

The methods utilized will be based on the paradigm of natural and traditional healing. The tools we will employ will be non-invasive, such as Dao yin exercises, diet, herbs, meditation, massage, qigong, Taijiquan, and specific remedies designed to heal any abnormalities, including diet and nutrition, and drugs. We will focus on a variety of causes and solutions.

Main Goal and Objectives

Our goal is for each and every person to recognize that they can heal, be healthy and, live well. First, we will start where you are. We will use education, observation, questions and analysis to determine if we can make a difference in your life. We will start where you are and will treat every person as an individual and total person.

Goals:

Be Healthy
Heal Your Life
Change Life
Live Well
Reduce, Eliminate or Prevent NCD's (Non-Communicable Diseases)

Objectives we will follow:

1.   Join the Healing Project
We invite all of you to join us
If you want to support us
If you need help or assistance
If you are interested in living well

2.   Determine where you are
Check to see if you are doing all you need or can to live well

Do you want to know what to do to improve your wellbeing?

3.   Determine what you need
To determine what you can do to change your life and become more balanced or healthy

4.   Determine any imbalances
We will do assessments to determine if you are in or out of balance

5.   Determine how to correct any imbalances
We will create a prescription, course of study, or a protocol to correct any imbalances
How to become balanced
Create a plan to provide solutions

6.   We will help one understand these concepts:

- What is health
- What is living well
- What is balance
- How to heal
- How to live well by changing our daily lives and what we do or don't do to maintain health and wellbeing

In Conclusion:

Are you ready? Then join us in becoming a part of "The Healing Project" and change your life, heal yourself and help us to heal others and pass the word on to the entire planet. So, ask yourself, how can we help you to live well, and how can you help others?

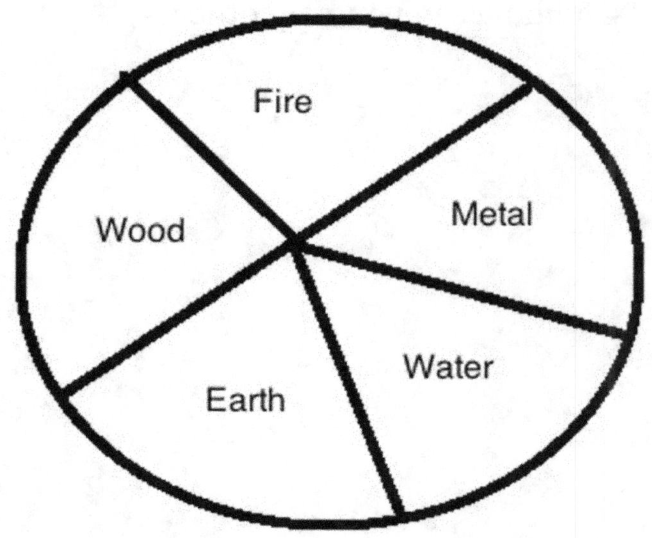

Five Elements Theory

Traditional Chinese medicine (TCM) is based on the philosophy of the yin-yang theory and the combination of the Five Phases theory, also called the Five Elements, which was later absorbed by Daoism. Five Elements is critical to the normal balance of the body and explains how nature is represented in human beings. The items in the Five Elements explain the connection of each element to the internal organs within the body and their corresponding connection to nature.

What is Missing?

The question is, what is missing with most people? It is how to stay healthy, and heal oneself; not just to survive, but also to live well. The answer is knowledge of self!

Many take health and healing for granted, assuming it will take care of itself. We wake up and expect to be healthy. We go about our business and play sports, running and jumping expecting that youth is another word for health and that throughout our adulthood, we are going to be healthy no matter what we do or don't do, or what we eat or don't eat, or how we treat ourselves.   It is ok to think we are healthy and to know it is important to think we are healthy. At the same time, we need to understand what is health, how to be healthy, how to stay healthy and how to heal ourselves. Being healthy and knowing what will keep us healthy is tantamount to healing ourselves day to day, or on a daily basis.

Yes, maintaining our health is a daily requirement and should never be ignored.

We get we are busy, but we should never be too busy to take care of our health and to learn how to be healthy and how to maintain our health. And, to heal ourselves, if required. So, if this is true, what is missing? Does everyone get this or know exactly what they need to know? Are they practicing it, or is it ignored until there is a problem or crisis? First for many, what is missing is the exact knowledge or critical information vital or necessary to accomplish the enormous task of being and maintaining one's health. In "The Healing Project" we hope to provide this missing knowledge that one can add and use to maintain their health, and live well. The second thing missing is how to change our life from one of sheer survival to one of living well.

We grow up with grandiose ideas of what we want to accomplish, watching TV shows about those who have everything at their fingertips, and think to ourselves, I will do and be that also. We then encounter the rest of the human race and find life is different than TV; we learn what our parents did not explain and realize that, sooner or later, we must survive like the beginner swimmer in the deep end of the pool. Joking around about life becomes serious quite soon, and then we have obligations that require us to put away the toys and get to work. And, sometimes, this pushes us and our health and wellbeing to the backburner, or to an obscure environment that we forget is important, as we chase the proverbial carrot that may or may not be healthy for us, all in the name of, "I am just trying to survive." Then, we wake up one day realizing that, in the race, we just survived, and our dream or goal of living well is a fantasy or made-for-TV movie, a the-rich-and-the-famous, crime-does-pay drama, in full HD 1080p.

*"A 90-year-old woman revealed how
she lives her best life.
Her biggest piece of advice is
simply to 'start with what you have.'
She also reveals she dances for two
hours each day and has a boyfriend she
exchanges books with."*
edinuzzo@businessinsider.com (Emily DiNuzzo)

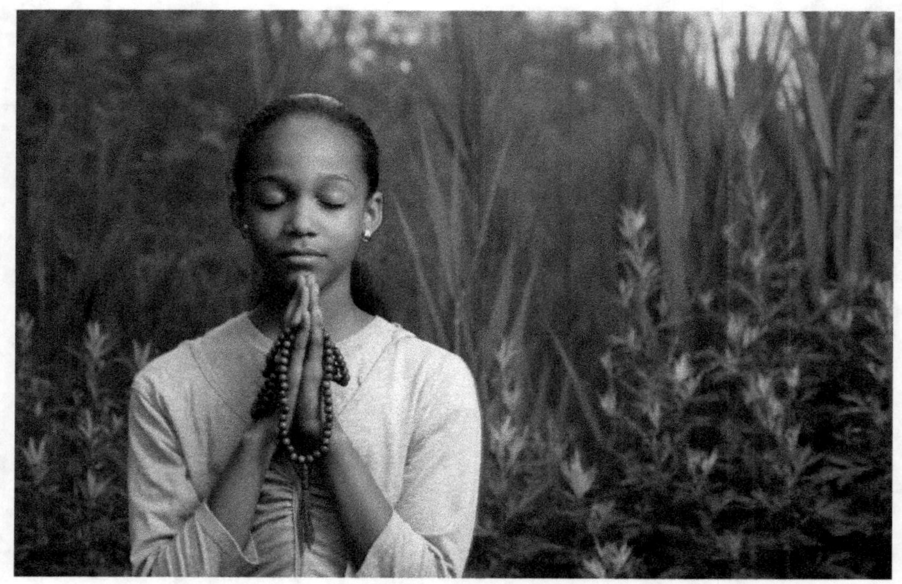

Who Am I

Our First Step

So, the first step is to know yourself. HOW DO I DO THAT? I thought I knew me, and everything in its totality. Well, maybe you do, or maybe you don't. Let's find out. How do we start? The first step is analysis, an overview, questions and answers, then a deeper analysis, more questions and answers. Then, a deeper understanding and revelation to determine if there is a consensus of what we know and don't know. Then, a 'where do we go from here.' Do we need information, more knowledge on a general or more specific subject matter? We consequently look at the total picture "wholistically", breaking down the different sectors we need to address. From there, we can assess what is there, what is missing, what is needed or what is not needed, and then develop a specific program for our individual self. This will include the sharing of knowledge that will help us to be healthy, heal and subsequently live well, as a direct or indirect result from our participation in "The Healing Project."

II

The Whole Person Versus a Section of a Person

When a person walks into the doctor's office, they bring with them the "whole person," not a part. If my arm is hurting or there is a pain in my foot, the doctor focuses on the part that appears to be in trouble at that moment. Sometimes that pain is not real, but only an appearance that there is something wrong or out of balance. Some prescribe pain medicine and then send the client home. To forego the Doctor, many people just go to the drug store and buy over the counter pain medicine and treat themselves. Many times, this works, and the pain is smothered or buffered and the feeling of pain is temporarily diminished or extinguished in a short time. This appears to work, so many people think that when there is pain, one just takes pain medication and that is the solution to the problem, until the pain increases and becomes unbearable. This then requires a Doctor or a trip to the hospital to receive stronger medication to quell the pain, or until the hospital realizes it is something greater and does tests to determine the cause of the pain. If the cause can be determined, then action is taken to correct the problem so the pain will recede. Sometimes this requires passive or invasive means to correct the problem. This can be the answer, or it can be only a temporary stopgap to alleviate the pain but not determine or correct the root cause to permanently correct the situation. The answer may lie in focusing on the total "whole person" to determine the root cause and then decide what is the best method to correct the problem and bring the person into a state of homeostasis, or balance. Too many times, people think the problem is gone or the crisis is over, only to have it come back again and again. This is because the root cause was never addressed; only temporary solutions were implemented, and the issue will continue until the cause is discovered and eliminated.

In traditional medicine the person was treated to determine the root cause and then how to correct the problem. In traditional or currently called "alternative medicine," one has to look beyond the mere external pain or problem to the root cause and try to determine if the so-called problem is masking something that the client or patient has not revealed or noticed. By first exploring the whole person, it is possible to determine the real cause of the problem and not focus on the pseudo cause. Focusing the treatment on the symptom and not the cause will temporarily alleviate the problem, but won't correct it permanently. This will cause the problem to return and never heal, which is an issue many people experience. When this happens, many people get frustrated and think their problem cannot be healed or corrected, and then they sometimes just settle for the medication as a way to manage their problem and give up on seeking the real solution. Managing the pain or situation does not fix the problem permanently but puts many people into survival mode, where they seek to just be able to survive in pain each and every day while TV commercials reinforce the ability to take 6-hour, 12-hour or 24-hour medication. They use the drug like it is food or nutrition, which it is not. Discounting the side effects is a disservice to the person taking the medication, because the side effects can be mild to very harmful, adding another dimension to the problem one already is experiencing.

So, in any health or healing situation the best way to help one's self or others is to focus on the whole person and determine if there are extenuating circumstances and the real cause. Once the root cause is determined, then one can figure out what is the best course of action to permanently remove the problem with the right solution and to make that person well and whole again. The question is, how to look at the whole person? For example, I treated a person who was very sick and had several very serious problems and was on various medications. I was asked if I could help. I did not look at the various problems or dis-eases or the medications she was taking. I asked her about whom she hated and held grudges against. Her answer was her ex-husband, who she had not seen in many years. I then first prescribed for her 3 ways to let go of the hatred and the grudges. Then, I recommended she come back in three months after she completed the three tasks. She went home and completed the tasks and then returned in three months to tell me that her health had improved and she was coming off some of her medications and some of the dosages were being cut in half. After six months, her health had improved and she was happy that her health was returning. The doctors that prescribed her the medications did not look at the whole person to see what triggered the decline in her health. They just focused on the symptoms and prescribed the medications that could temporarily provide relief for her problems. They did what they were trained to do in modern medicine. This is why in traditional medicine is different, because everything the person does contributes to the whole being; and as a medical practitioner, one must look at the total person in order to remove any causes so that a person can heal permanently.

In Conclusion

One must consider the whole person, body, mind and spirit, to understand what is required. Managing a problem is different than solving a problem or providing a solution. Part of living well and healthy is to do so on a body, mind, and spirit level, not just one piece. We do not want to only consider a piece, but the total package. In the "The Health Project," we will endeavor to look at and consider the whole person. If there is a problem, we will try and determine the root cause and then correct this cause to provide a total and permanent solution, if at all possible. From there, we are able to stay in balance and maintain our health and wellbeing. Living well requires us to consider the whole person holistically, beyond their physical health.

III

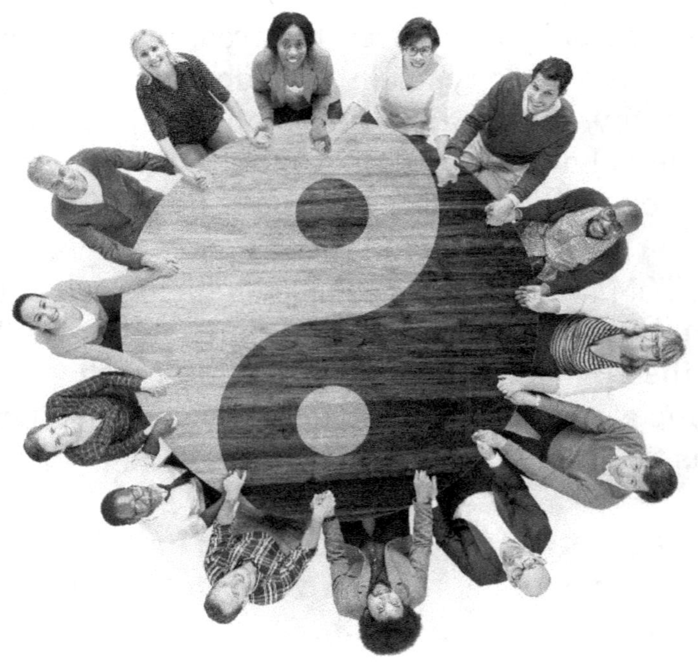

Good Family Health

What is Health?

What is health? Health is defined as the state of being free of illness and injury. What is holistic health? Holistic health is a diverse field of medicine that focuses on the total or whole person. It is important to understand this in its entirety. What is modern medicine? Modern medicine is considered the scientific treatment of prevention of disease utilizing non-invasive and invasive methods and drugs. What is alternative medicine? Alternative medicine is sometimes known as "complementary" or "holistic" medicine. There is a long list of what alternative medicine actually comprises, but treatments falling under the umbrella typically include acupuncture, homeopathy, chiropractic, herbal medicine, Reiki, laying on of hands, energy or sound therapy, meditation, massage, aromatherapy, hypnosis, Ayurveda (a traditional medical practice originating in India), TCM (Traditional Chinese Medicine originating in China) and several other treatments not normally prescribed by mainstream doctors. Alternative medicine is considered to be non-invasive medicine. What is traditional medicine? Traditional medicine is considered or named as indigenous or folk medicine comprised of knowledge systems that have been developed over generations from various societies and/or cultures before the development of modern medicine.

What does the total or whole person include?

The whole or total person includes the physical, mental, psychological, energetic and spiritual aspects of a person. All of these above attributes sum up the total or whole person. The health is within you, and around you there is Nature, which is here to help you to be and stay healthy. There are many physical and mental processes to assist you in being healthy, including spiritual processes, which give us universal assistance. These advise us to know we are healthy, and it is within us to maintain that health and to live well to stay healthy. When we look in the mirror, we see a healthy image, and all we do should include maintaining that healthy image. If there is a problem, we should begin to correct ourselves so our image reflects our health within ourselves and externally. The universe and Nature supports us, and we support ourselves in living well by taking good care of families and ourselves. In modern society, some are looking away from nature and are looking toward science as the panacea. A lot of this science is the introduction and proliferation of drugs. Some now think everything is in the drugs or the genetic engineering of foods and chemicals, including the use of surgery and surgical modifications. So many do not know where to turn. They say, should I be traditional, or turn toward science, which is touted as the miracle? What should I do? I say, be traditional with some assistance when required from the science community when it is safe. First, educate yourself, then, make the best decisions with the idea of insuring that the total person is included and the cause and effect is addressed. One should focus on solutions and not just management. And remember, addiction is not a cure.

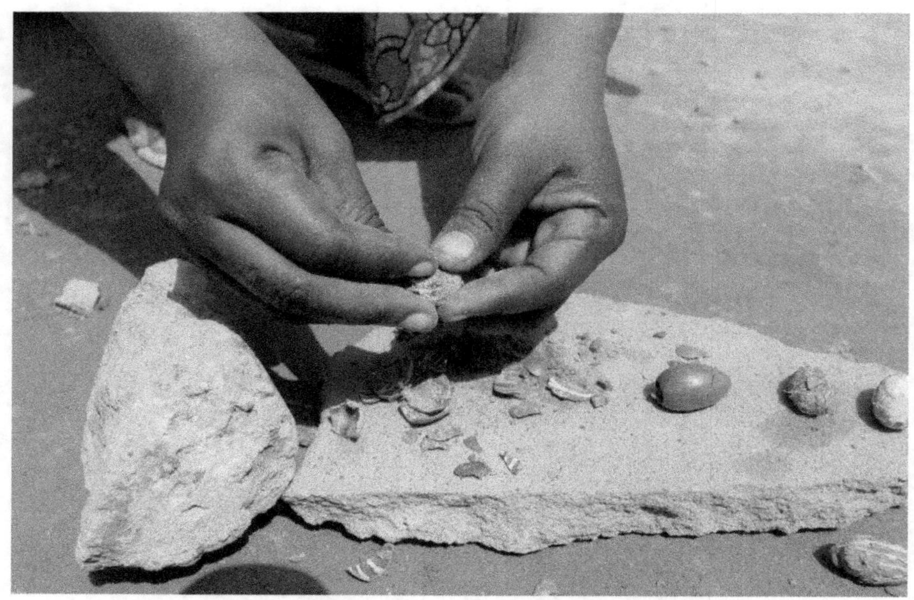

Natural Medicine

Is Health in the Drugs or Nature?

A great question, is health in the drugs? Well, if not why are drugs prescribed so much for everything from keeping awake, to going to sleep, to children growing up?

This is an important question because in the Western world, many rely heavily on drugs as a panacea to good or great health. Steroids are almost worshipped, and pain medication may be considered a daily food just as caffeine is tantamount to the universal elixir. Diet drugs are like watching people on TV exercise and you receiving the benefit. The words "good old fashioned" and "traditional" are being thrown out for "new and improved" or "genetically engineered." Lawyers are getting rich off of so-called "bad drugs" once deemed great or good or the next best thing. The new verbiage is it will either heal you or kill you when qualifying some drugs as the ultimate in healing. If you are solely relying on a drug, you are surviving and not living well. But let us not forget that some drugs are necessary, do help us, and so we cannot condemn all drugs. It is not our intention to do so, but to shine a light and realize that we want to be healed and not addicted or controlled by some outside force like the power of some drugs, which can also be detrimental to our overall good health and wellbeing.

Nature, on the other hand, provides all the drugs one needs, but the drugs are in the form of foods and herbs that have little or no side effects that are detrimental to one's health. Natural medicine is considered traditional and not modern or scientific. The natural medicine is for human beings, but some think that medicine has to be scientific, even though the litany of side effects has proven detrimental to the overall health of some individuals. The western world thinks that science has all the answers, but there are too many unanswered questions.

IV

Modern Medicine and the Case for Drugs

There are more than 24,000 drugs, and drugs have helped many people, just as drugs that have caused a multitude of problems have hurt many people. This comes from one of the criteria listed below:

Overdose
Wrong medication
Allergic reaction to certain drugs
Bad drugs
Bad compounding drugs
Sicknesses from side effects
Side effects creating other dis-eases
Placebo drugs
Bogus drugs from Black Market
Poisonous drugs

"This situation means that, right now, *prescription drugs are killing 100,000 Americans each year and injuring more than two million*. Those are the statistics from the Journal of the American Medical Association, and that figure doesn't include the 40,000 or so who are killed each year by over-the-counter pain medications." This doesn't include drug dependence and addiction.

What More is Needed to Wake You Up?

Do you need to be hit in the head with an empty bottle of harmful drugs? What more information is required for one to wakeup and see that drugs have side effects that are sometimes not conducive to healing, and the side effects may be worse than the initial problem and prognosis? Taking the wrong prescribed medicine can produce very negative results. Many drugs are addictive. Some drugs have dangerous ingredients. So, what does one do, is the question many ask. The answer may be to research natural and non-chemical drug solutions. Ask the question, will holistic medicine provide any solutions? Are there non-invasive solutions that should be explored first? Should one focus on finding the cause of their problem or disease, or just take a pill that may only mask the problem and not provide a complete solution. I talked to a teacher who was taking a drug for depression, and all she did was cry all the time. It was wrecking her life and work. She came to me to find out what was the problem and was shocked when I told her it was the pills she was taking. Once she stopped the pills, the crying stopped, and she was able to return to normalcy and focus on what was making her upset (her husband). Another case I handled was with a lady who was getting very sick from taking prescribed pills for a problem that was not even there. The pills made her internal system (liver and kidneys) toxic, and I recommended she stop the pills and take some herbs and to drink a lot of water. She followed my instructions and her husband explained that for the next few weeks, the toxicity was pouring out of her body and smelled up their home until the detox was finished. After that, she was better and back in balance and healthy. There are countless stories.

Is Sickness and Dis-ease Diminishing or Growing?

Has anyone noticed that, in the modern world, there appears to be an increase in longevity and an increase in sickness? Have you asked yourself if dis-ease has increased, or are the newspapers and TV lying? Or are there extenuating circumstances surrounding the general health and wellbeing of people in the world today?

*This extract taken from the website Healthy Secrets states: **"In these days of so called medical enlightenment infectious diseases are killing the world at the rate of 1,500 deaths per hour! Yet even more so are what are considered as non-infectious diseases: cancer and heart disease. Though new evidence shows that these diseases may indeed have infectious causes. Topping these are medical mistakes! These are the true top killers decimating families faster than anything else in this world."***

Most people do not realize that in their desire to beat the illness, they succumb to even more dangerous prescription drugs and medical practices. Deaths from prescription drugs are escalating rapidly. Even dis-ease names are deceptive and appear to be designed to confuse patients about cause, prevention and treatment. Clearly the fastest way to be healed is to establish cause and effect AS SOON AS POSSIBLE. Doctors usually give the party line that they do not know what is causing your sickness! If that is true, then does logic not tell you that this failure to identify the true cause of a disease results in an incorrect judgment of what must be done to correct it? Ultimately, zero cases are actually permanently 'cured' with our modern day advanced treatments.

Every day, we live to heal ourselves with nutritious foods or ingesting foods that do the opposite, but it is our choice. We choose to smoke cigarettes or not, we choose to ingest harmful drugs or not, or we can choose to make sure that we do not harm our bodies with contaminants. Part of eating to live is to try and not eat those foods that are harmful to our health and wellbeing. Farmers once wanted us to have nutritious foods, but it seems that the modern corporate approach to maximum profits uses chemicals, scientific tricks, and any means to maximize profits, while at the same time, adding chemicals to our foods and soil is causing problems instead of making sure our foods are more nutritious. If the description of the side effects of some drugs, are longer and more complicated than the actual drug, one should try and reconsider what is the best course of action and if there are any positive alternatives.

List of Dangerous Drugs to the Body from Side Effects
"From herbs-info.com"

1 Sleeping pills
2 Cholesterol drugs
3 Blood pressure drugs
4 Alzheimer drugs
5 Arthritis drugs
6 Diabetes drugs
7 Chemotherapy drugs

"This above list is from a Harvard report from the European Commission that ranks dangerous the 4th highest cause of death. This is important we are not saying you should not take these drugs prescribed by your doctor but you should know the risks to your life before ingesting these drugs."

One More Thing to Consider

How does the food you eat affect your body and your life, and how does food work with the medications you are taking? Some foods intensify your medications, and some foods interfere with the medications you take. Some foods, when coupled with the medications you are taking, can be harmful to you, so you must be aware of what to eat and what to avoid when taking certain medications. For example, grapefruit can interfere with certain statin drugs for high cholesterol. Or, eating foods such as bananas when taking blood pressure drugs is not advisable and can be harmful. Research your medications and foods that adversely affect each other.

In Conclusion

If drugs cause dangerous side effects or are detrimental to our overall health, we should consider alternatives. If drugs are addictive and cause us to now have to survive with the drug in order to live with an addition, we should again consider alternatives that are not so controlling or health destroying. If a drug has poisonous ingredients, we should consider alternatives that are more homogenous to our overall health and wellbeing. If drugs takeover our internal health system and control it, we should explore more holistic solutions that can heal and not control us. Drugs should be categorized by their ability to heal, level of addiction, side effects, damage to our life and the ability to totally heal us before being administered as a miracle or panacea or even safe for human consumption. I want to know if this drug can heal me or just manage or control me, or shorten or lengthen my life. Do I want to live or just survive, ask yourself? What is this drug doing to my life and my goal of living well?

Mistake Over Now Pill Free

Making a mistake
I took the fake pill
It did not save me
But it made me
Realize the pain is in the pill
My cells it did kill
Good and bad
It is sad
I was healthy
Before I had
This pill
That made me ill
I take it everyday
Now I have become a crook
Because I am hooked
On the pain that is making me insane
For I cannot afford the pills anymore
And I swore
I will not take them anymore
Because they are in my core
Now they are in control
And I am in the hole
To the doctor that did prescribe
The best high I can describe
And then no pain
All is gone
My money
My health
My fame
For others see
That it is not me
But the pill that walks the street
As if I am ill
But I am only sick of these pills
And can't stop

Since they have taken control
Of my bank
And my funds have sank
Into oblivion and I am worn
So I can morn the day I stop
These drugs or they stop me
Cold no more sold
Over the counter
Or under the table
Because now I am stable
Save the day
Save the children
Wave the flag
For all to stop
Adopt the herb
Eat the food
And take the time
To heal all of me
Not just the bruise you see
But the cause that is key
Problem solved
And now I am pill free.

V

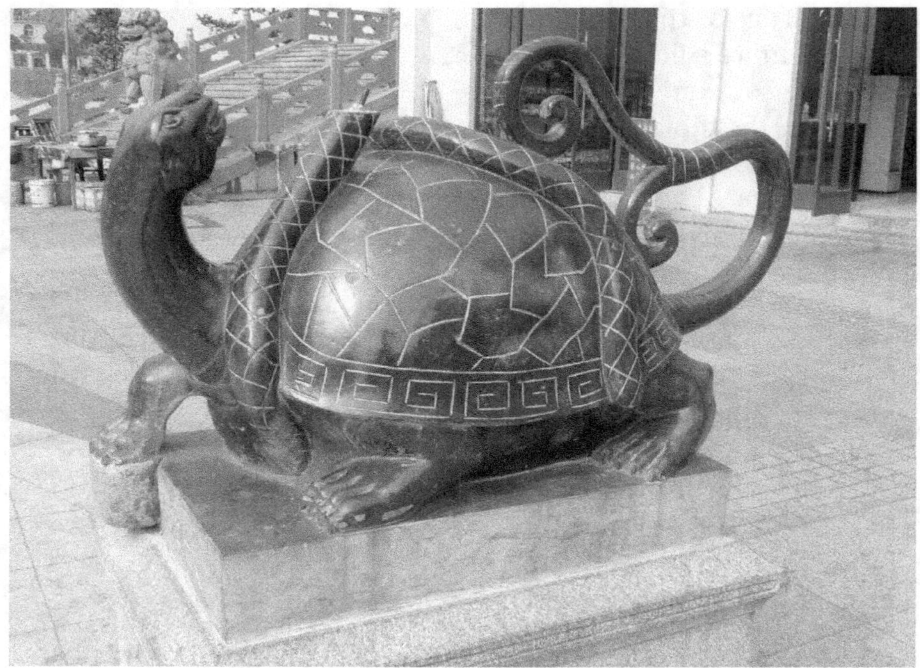

Long Life Tortoise

What is Life?

Life is the condition that distinguishes animals and plants from inorganic matter, including the capacity for growth, reproduction, functional activity, and continual change preceding death. Life is also the existence of an individual human being or animal or anything that is alive and breathing.

What is life about?

Life is about living through that period between the birth and death of a living thing, an organism or a human being.

What do we do everyday?

We live each and every day alive, being and doing whatever it is that we do through breathing and any functional activities that we do on a daily basis.

Can we live our life as we want to?

Yes we can if we elect to do so. We can live full of life and with everything that life brings us.

Do we live life, or do we just survive?

We live life everyday and make our decisions based on surviving or living well as we choose to do and be.

Do we take life for granted?

Some take life for granted because life is granted to us due to the fact we are alive, but do we take health for granted is the better question. That is a yes also, but we should not take it too lightly since part of our job is to maintain our life and health.

Do we struggle, or do we just live?

Some of us live well from being granted a life well planned by parents, while others struggle and everything is not handed to them. Others struggle just to get used to life as it is in our local environment, and those around us that make life easy or a struggle.

How are you living?

Are you living well, or just surviving and is all well or just a struggle? Ask yourself how you are living. This will help us to live a long, fruitful life or to struggle, or something in between.

What Factors Shorten Life

These are the most dangerous factors that can cause the shortening of life. These factors can have an adverse effect on you, but the good news is that, once known, you can change the paradigm and correct any of these factors that are affecting you and your longevity. Nothing on this list is difficult to understand.

o   Sleep Deprivation: go to bed at night, take naps, staying up all day and night is not wise
o   Dehydration: drink water, and soda is not water
o   Physical Fitness: exercise each day, even if only for a short period, especially if you are retired
o   Stupidity: smarten up, wise up, and being stubborn is not a virtue
o   Lack of Using Brainpower: use it, it's not just for wearing a hat

- o Environmental Toxicity: smoke, fumes, chemicals, poison, asbestos, and pesticides need attention and cleaning up
- o Harmful Drugs: using and overdosing on illegal and legal drugs
- o Stress: related to tension, worry, anxiety and fear for whatever reasons; let go
- o Shootings: people and cops with guns kill people
- o Wars: warmongers perpetrate endless wars; going to war is not a job!
- o Lack of activity: get moving
- o Smoking cigarettes
- o Bad, processed foods

What Factors Help to Increase Long Life

- o Spiritual consciousness
- o Calmness and Peace
- o Satisfaction with less or more
- o Lack of external societal tension and stress
- o Active life
- o Lifelong learning and mental stimulation
- o Nutrition
- o Energy
- o Belief
- o Good Relationships
- o Minimizing stress and tension

Effects

What affects different areas of the body system, and how do you support and repair them? How do they affect our life, longevity, living healthy, and well?

Metabolism- the chemical processes that occur within a living organism in order to maintain life-requires movement of external and internal systems. Too much non-movement is not good.

Digestion- Digestion is the breakdown of large insoluble food molecules into small water-soluble food molecules so that they can be absorbed into the watery blood plasma. In certain organisms, these smaller substances are absorbed through the small intestine into the blood stream. The ability to digest whatever one eats is a requirement.

Elimination- the expulsion of waste matter from the body: the moving out of stuff within our system that needs to be eliminated requires movement of the body through exercises.

Lymphatic system- is part of the circulatory system and a vital part of the immune system, comprising a network of lymphatic vessels that carry a clear fluid called lymph directionally towards the heart. We must keep it clear and moving.

Energetic system- Energy is required for all kinds of bodily processes including growth and development, repair, the transport of various substances, between cells, and of course, muscle contraction. This includes different types of energy such as pre-natal and postnatal energies that keep us alive, strong and healthy. We get energy from the Earth, Sun, Universe, foodstuffs and herbs.

Physical muscles- Physical exercise is any bodily activity that enhances or maintains physical fitness and overall health and wellness. Muscles keep our bodies moving and strong non-exercise is not good-exercise and movement is required.

Tendons- tendon or sinew is a tough band of fibrous connective tissue that usually connects muscle to bone and is capable of withstanding tension. Tendons are similar to ligaments; both are made of collagen. Ligaments join one bone to another bone, while tendons connect muscle to bone-exercise is vital.

Ligaments- In anatomy, a ligament is the fibrous connective tissue that connects bones to other bones and is also known as articular ligament, articular cartilage, fibrous ligament, or true ligament. These hold our bodies and joints together and provide elasticity within our internal system-exercise and stretching is vital.

Breathing System- The process of taking air into the lungs is called inhalation or inspiration, and the process of breathing it out is called exhalation or expiration. Breathing, which keeps one alive, brings in oxygen and energy from the air, which is used to oxygenate our blood to feed our internal systems. Breathing is vital so try to practice deep breathing everyday.

Brain system- is part of the nervous system is your body's decision and communication center. The central nervous system (CNS) is made of the brain and the spinal cord, and the peripheral nervous system (PNS) is made of nerves. The brain runs the body system and requires oxygen and essential nutrients and proper stimulation- mental and intellectual stimulation, is also required.

Balance system-our internal systems must be in balance, especially our energetic and mental systems-relaxation and centeredness is required to release stress and worry.

Circulation system- the circulatory system, also called the cardiovascular system or the vascular system, is an organ system that permits blood to circulate and transport nutrients (such as amino acids and electrolytes), oxygen, carbon dioxide, hormones, and blood cells to and from the cells in the body to provide nourishment and help in fighting diseases, stabilize temperature and pH, and maintaining homeostasis. Our blood, nutrients, oxygen, hormones and energies must circulate to keep us healthy–exercise is important, as well as activity.

Blood pressure system-is a part of the circulatory system- Hypertension is the medical term for high blood pressure. Blood pressure must be in balance also to keep our internal systems under control, to insure our internal system is running at optimum. Water is required and not too much ingestion of salt

Strength system-muscles, tendons, ligaments, bones and internal energy must be strong-exercise and activity is required.

Longevity system-we must keep our internal and external systems running at optimum to be able to live long and live well.

Joints systems-also known as articulations, they are strong connections that join the bones, teeth, and cartilage of the body to one another. Each joint is specialized in its shape and structural components to control the range of motion between the parts that it connects to. They must be in good health, fluid and free moving so we are at a flexible point without blocks and stiffness-movement and stretching is important.

Growth system-our internal growth system keeps us growing from blood, to bone to cells and hormones along with our energy. Movement and exercise is important, as is the ingestion and digestion of essential nutrients from our diets.

Effects of Abuses

Abuse is a subject that is not discussed in mixed company because the definition speaks to how many people experience their life and the suffering they deal with on a daily basis. Some people work in abusive environments that cause a great deal of stress in their lives. Abuses can stem very many avenues such as the abuse of alcohol, to illegal and legal drugs, to the abuse of food, mental abuses of relationships, the police, sexual, war, racism and many more avenues than can be discussed here. These abuses lead to causes of non-communicable dis-eases and need to be mitigated, eliminated or managed in a way that they do not affect the health and welfare of people who are affected each and everyday of their lives. Why you ask as you try to get your head around this statement, stress and tension caused by abuses lead to hypertension and other dis-eases. Stress for example, is the leading cause of most problems with the brain-mind connection, the heart-mind connection and many other problems with the mind-body connections.

Some abuses are in categories:

Self-afflicted
Willfully impressed upon others
Unknowingly caused by their environment
Caused by the government policies
Human behavior
Lack of knowledge or information
Access to proper healthcare
Over indulgence
Lack of balance
Misunderstandings
Deprivation

In Conclusion

Abuses are important to understand since many problems experienced in society affect large populations such as poverty, caused by government polices such as homelessness or a lack of government policies that support people and their communities. Self affliction is a huge problems because of stuff like drug addiction that can be self afflicted or willfully impressed on others by outside forces such as medicinal drugs that lead to drug addiction and end destroying large populations of families. Many abuses are connected such as drug addiction and over indulgence, which is connected to human behavior. Lack of information is causing innumerable problems because many people do not understand what they are doing to their bodies and they're minds, and how each affects each other. The body and brain-mind are not lone soldiers operating outside of each other. Poverty is causing major problems since there are multiple problems with proper nutrition, deprivation, and lack of access to proper healthcare. So abuses are connected to the causes of non-communicable dis-eases and the ability to prevent and reduce NCDs since the majority populations suffering from NCDs are communities of poverty, disadvantaged and exclusion from proper information and healthcare. Abusive behavior like overindulgence or bad habits is attributed to causal effects of a variety of NCDs. when abuses are eliminated it will help reduce NCDs and improve the overall health and wellbeing of many people.

Short List of Non-communicable Dis-eases (NCDs)

This short list of NCDs can be prevented with education and information about diet, exercise, the elimination of bad habits such as smoking, too many sweets, or too much salt, water dehydration, proper rest, chemical pollutants, environmental toxicity, and early detection.

1. Diabetes

2. Hypertension

3. Osteoporosis

4. Alzheimer's

5. Heart Disease

6. Fibromyalgia

7. Lung Cancer

8. Leukemia

9. Skin Cancer

10. Seizures or Epilepsy

In Conclusion

These internal and external systems must be kept in good condition so that we can remain healthy, live long and live well without getting sick from NCDs that will limit our lifestyle, and our goal of living well. One thing that is very clear is that one needs to keep moving and doing. The effects we have on these systems to keep them at optimum require us to exercise regularly, feed ourselves nutrients properly, and get proper rest.

How to Reduce, Prevent or Eliminate (Non-Communicable Dis-eases)

What facilities or methods will help you to be healthy and live well at any age and prevent non-communicable dis-eases? There are several methods. This includes physical and mental remedies. The importance of exercise as a healing art to help in the prevention of NCDs is one way. Understanding the causes of NCDs is another. A third is through the traditional (alternative) healing arts.

More about NCDs is explained below in the World Health Organization's extract below.

Extract from WHO: Key facts

Noncommunicable diseases (NCDs) kill 40 million people each year, equivalent to 70% of all deaths globally.

Each year, 15 million people die from a NCD between the ages of 30 and 69 years; over 80% of these "premature" deaths occur in low- and middle-income countries.

Cardiovascular diseases account for most NCD deaths, or 17.7 million people annually, followed by cancers (8.8 million), respiratory diseases (3.9million), and diabetes (1.6 million).

These 4 groups of diseases account for over 80% of all premature NCD deaths.

Tobacco use, physical inactivity, the harmful use of alcohol and unhealthy diets all increase the risk of dying from a NCD.

Detection, screening and treatment of NCDs, as well as palliative care, are key components of the response to NCDs.

Overview
Noncommunicable diseases (NCDs), also known as chronic diseases, tend to be of long duration and are the result of a combination of genetic, physiological, environmental and behaviors factors.

The main types of NCDs are cardiovascular diseases (like heart attacks and stroke), cancers, chronic respiratory diseases (such as chronic obstructive pulmonary disease and asthma) and diabetes.

NCDs disproportionately affect people in low- and middle-income countries where more than three quarters of global NCD deaths – 31 million – occur.

Who is at risk of such diseases?
People of all age groups, regions and countries are affected by NCDs. These conditions are often associated with older age groups, but evidence shows that 15 million of all deaths attributed to NCDs occur between the ages of 30 and 69 years. Of these "premature" deaths, over 80% are estimated to occur in low- and middle-income countries. Children, adults and the elderly are all vulnerable to the risk factors contributing to NCDs, whether from unhealthy diets, physical inactivity, exposure to tobacco smoke or the harmful use of alcohol.

These diseases are driven by forces that include rapid unplanned urbanization, globalization of unhealthy lifestyles and population ageing. Unhealthy diets and a lack of physical activity may show up in people as raised blood pressure, increased blood glucose, elevated blood lipids and obesity. These are called metabolic risk factors that can lead to cardiovascular disease, the leading NCD in terms of premature deaths.

Risk factors
Modifiable behavioral risk factors
Modifiable behaviors, such as tobacco use, physical inactivity, unhealthy diet and the harmful use of alcohol, all increase the risk of NCDs.

> *Tobacco accounts for 7.2 million deaths every year (including from the effects of exposure to second-hand smoke), and is projected to increase markedly over the coming years. (1)*
> *4.1 million annual deaths have been attributed to excess salt/sodium intake. (1)*
> *More than half of the 3.3 million annual deaths attributable to alcohol use are from NCDs, including cancer. (2)*
> *1.6 million deaths annually can be attributed to insufficient physical activity. (1)*

Metabolic risk factors
Metabolic risk factors contribute to four key metabolic changes that increase the risk of NCDs:

- *raised blood pressure*
- *overweight/obesity*
- *hyperglycemia (high blood glucose levels) and*
- *hyperlipidemia (high levels of fat in the blood).*

In terms of attributable deaths, the leading metabolic risk factor globally is elevated blood pressure (to which 19% of global deaths are attributed), (1) followed by overweight and obesity and raised blood glucose.

What are the socioeconomic impacts of NCDs?

NCDs threaten progress towards the 2030 Agenda for Sustainable Development, which includes a target of reducing premature deaths from NCDs by one-third by 2030.

Poverty is closely linked with NCDs. The rapid rise in NCDs is predicted to impede poverty reduction initiatives in low-income countries, particularly by increasing household costs associated with health care. Vulnerable and socially disadvantaged people get sicker and die sooner than people of higher social positions, especially because they are at greater risk of being exposed to harmful products, such as tobacco, or unhealthy dietary practices, and have limited access to health services.

In low-resource settings, health-care costs for NCDs quickly drain household resources. The exorbitant costs of NCDs, including often lengthy and expensive treatment and loss of breadwinners, force millions of people into poverty annually and stifle development.

Prevention and control of NCDs
An important way to control NCDs is to focus on reducing the risk factors associated with these diseases. Low-cost solutions exist for governments and other stakeholders to reduce the common modifiable risk factors. Monitoring progress and trends of NCDs and their risk is important for guiding policy and priorities.

To lessen the impact of NCDs on individuals and society, a comprehensive approach is needed requiring all sectors, including health, finance, transport, education, agriculture, planning and others, to collaborate to reduce the risks associated with NCDs, and promote interventions to prevent and control them.

Investing in better management of NCDs is critical. Management of NCDs includes detecting, screening and treating these diseases, and providing access to palliative care for people in need. High impact essential NCD interventions can be delivered through a primary health care approach to strengthen early detection and timely treatment. Evidence shows such interventions are excellent economic investments because, if provided early to patients, they can reduce the need for more expensive treatment.

Countries with inadequate health insurance coverage are unlikely to provide universal access to essential NCD interventions. NCD management interventions are essential for achieving the global target of a 25% relative reduction in the risk of premature mortality from NCDs by 2025, and the SDG target of a one-third reduction in premature deaths from NCDs by 2030.

WHO response
WHO's leadership and coordination role

The 2030 Agenda for Sustainable Development recognizes NCDs as a major challenge for sustainable development. As part of the Agenda, Heads of State and Government committed to develop ambitious national responses, by 2030, to reduce by one-third premature mortality from NCDs through prevention and treatment (SDG target 3.4). This target comes from the High-level Meetings of the UN General Assembly on NCDs in 2011 and 2014, which reaffirmed WHO's leadership and coordination role in promoting and monitoring global action against NCDs. The UN General Assembly will convene a third High-level Meeting on NCDs in 2018 to review progress and forge consensus on the road ahead covering the period 2018-2030.

To support countries in their national efforts, WHO developed a Global action plan for the prevention and control of NCDs 2013-2020, which includes nine global targets that have the

In Conclusion

Does this affect living well? Yes, we strive to live well and prevent non-communicable dis-eases (NCDs) that could affect us. This can be done, through creating programs of activities, early detection and exercises that will keep us healthy and balanced. This will prevent us from being affected by NCDs and will lead to our overall health, living longer and living well. Exercises are not just for certain people and not only for fun but also for keeping us in optimum health and achieving our goal of living well, and living longer. Exercise is one remedy, and meditation is another; correcting the diet, and stopping smoking, stopping worrying or stressing and healing the causes of the dis-ease are other methods. The problem should be attacked on physical, mental and spiritual levels holistically.

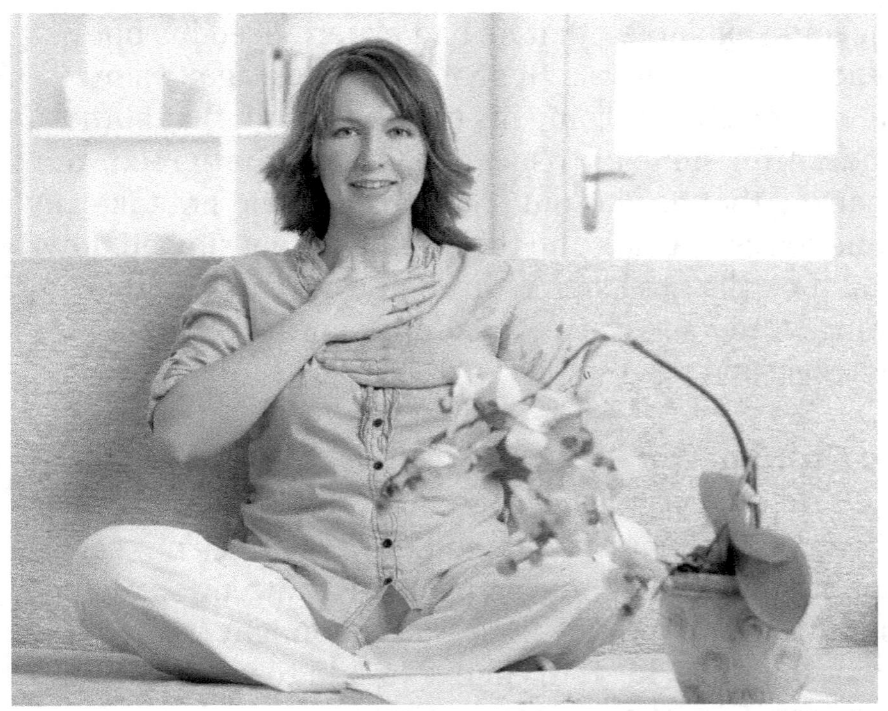

Self-Healing

What are We Paying Attention to?

What are you paying attention to; money, partying, animals sleeping in your bed, or your health? Who comes first, you, or everything else, then you and your health? Is anything more important to you? Or do you leave it up to the doctor and the hospital? I remember a story. I was talking to a friend of mine who was very rich, had the most beautiful wife and all the toys one could ask for. So he partied and ran the road 24/7, burning the proverbial candle at both ends. He was totally fit with a ripped body, but one day his bicep blew out. He wondered why this would happen to such a lucky guy with the best and perfect life. He queried me and I explained that he had experienced his body reaching burnout, and it sent him a message to slow down and stop burning his body (or candle) at both ends. After some introspective thought, he agreed, and realized that he was out of control and did not take any time to rest. Luckily, he then immediately slowed down and took time to listen to his body systems and to bring things into balance i.e. some fun, some work, some exercise and then some rest.

In Conclusion

Wealth cannot buy health and the body does not care about your wealth only its health. Pay attention, do not panic at what you see on the list that might trigger something you need to change or add to your daily regimen. Just ponder it and do what you feel you should do. Anything that can help you is always a good thing. Are you paying attention to your health? Are you living well? Do we need to hear the litany of lawyers on TV advertising about how to file lawsuits against pharmaceutical companies and hospitals for the prescription of bad or wrongful drug medication? Are you one of these or about to be? Is it more important to improve your health now or get assistance from Holistic Health Practitioners to help you heal naturally?

Some people never heal or are never in good health either by their own fault or circumstances out of their control. Do we stay status quo, do we change our thinking and begin to explore what we can do to improve our health and/or heal our own self, or do we

wait for the maid to cleanup only to realize we do not
have a maid and must clean up the house ourselves?
Even if you have a maid, she cannot give you her health.

VI

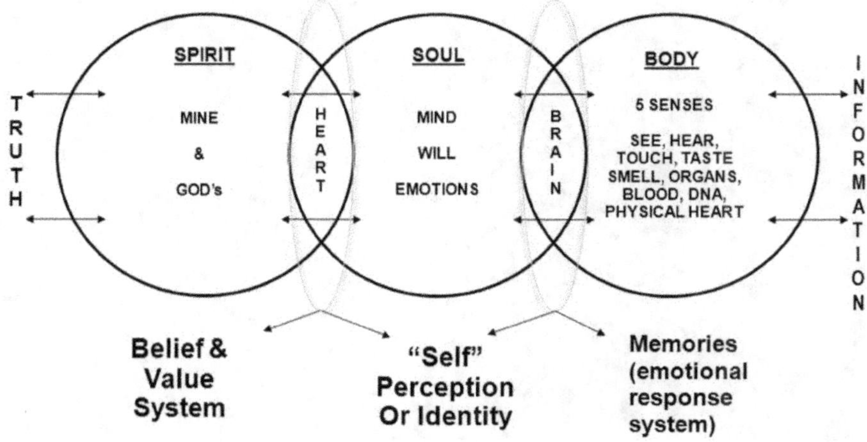

African Health Model

So Where Do We Begin?

So where do we begin? The answer is with you. Is it a medical checkup, a holistic checkup, or a total whole personal checkup that includes body, mind and soul? What is the difference? The medical checkup is a good place to start, and we all should get yearly checkups. At the same time, we should get a holistic checkup with a Holistic Practitioner once a year, or once every six months and whenever we feel the need or if we feel we are out of balance. Or, if there is a problem we are experiencing or any past problem(s) or issue(s) that have not been addressed sufficiently.

Information is key. So, let's start at understanding what is the meaning is of the term "healing." The term "healing ", is defined as the process of becoming sound, in balance or healthy again. What is a healer? A healer is a person that heals, or alleviates pain or distress of him or herself or another person. Another definition is a person who claims to be able to cure a disease or injury using special powers. These special powers can be a variety of skills or tools that address and consider the whole person.

So, if we focus on healing, then we have to first ask questions such as:

Can a person heal?

Yes, a person can heal. The body and mind has the ability to heal itself.

Can a person self-heal?

Yes, a person can self-heal, and it has been proven time and again, since 98 percent, of all healing is done by the person, all by themselves. The majority of the time, the body heals itself or warns the person that there is something that needs to be addressed or is out of balance. At first the body tries to correct the problem and simultaneously warns the person that something needs to be addressed whether we take notice or not. Most doctors will tell you that the body heals itself, and continues to heal itself, and that it triggers that it needs a person to pay attention, to stop causing a problem or out-of-balance condition. If not, sometimes the body will require outside assistance to bring attention to the problem that is affecting the body or the mind.

Can a person embark on a healing journey and actually make a difference in their overall health?

Yes, a person can change their overall health and cure or heal specific conditions. This is why one can change from unhealthy habits to healthy habits that will make a difference in their overall health. For example, many people realize smoking cigarettes is not good for their health, but some choose to ignore it while some health-conscious people realize the effect upon their health and change from smoking to non-smoking which helps to improve their health over time as the unhealthy smoke and nicotine is no longer there to affect their lungs, blood, and other internal organs. Over time, their body begins to clear itself of the toxicity and tries to heal any problems caused by the hazardous smoking habit. Another example, is how a person that uses too much sugar can cause problems to their system such as the person we have seen that needs six sugars in their cup of coffee or who drinks a lot of sweet tea and eats a lot of sweets. Sometimes this can affect their blood sugar balance but they can decide to stop using and ingesting so much sugar thereby helping the balance of the glucose in their system so that they will not suffer a diabetic condition. Fortunately, or unfortunately, we get most of the salt and sugar we need from the all the processed foods we buy everyday from the supermarket or restaurant.

Can a group create a project on health, and healing and significantly make a difference and achieve better health and wellness for all involved (themselves and others)?

We can all share what we learn from our own practice to improve our health and wellness, and share the good information and news with those who need and request our assistance. We can create an environment for others to participate and improve their health such as a walking group, or a Taijiquan group or yoga group, or a healing and wellness group.

In Conclusion

We can heal ourselves, and we can help others. We can change any unhealthy habits to healthy ones if we want to, simply by deciding that we want to improve our health, and wellness. Simply by changing our minds, to do so. We can create a program of change or learning what we can do to improve our own health. We can help ourselves even if we do not have access to health care because of costs or location. Poverty is not an excuse, and ignorance or lack of knowledge is not an adequate excuse. Access to information is available, as is access to health professionals to assist us if we desire it.

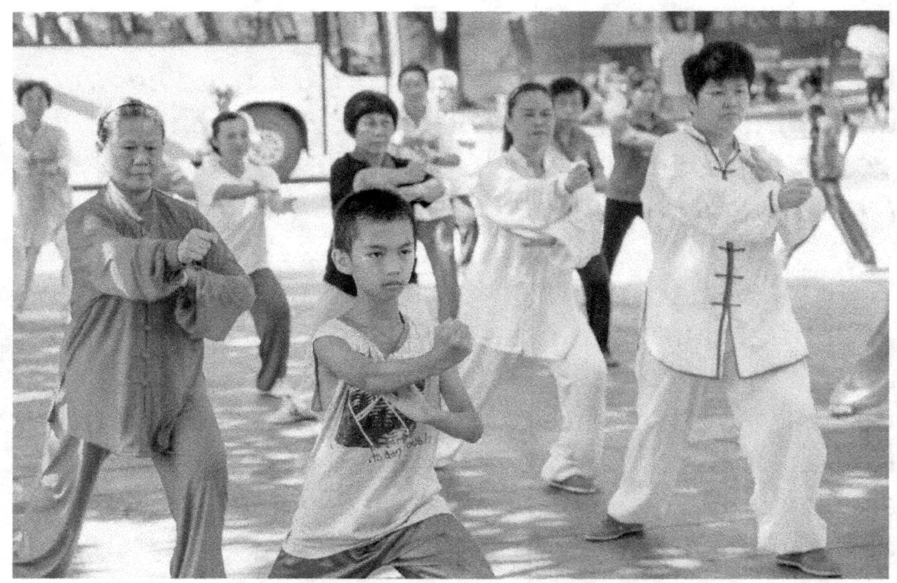

TaijiQuan Practice

How Do We Start?

There are two major paths. One is to begin by completing a general scan of the whole body and mind through basic screenings. The second is to start with what appears to ail a person and begin there, and then completing a whole person screening to determine the cause and what is happening to a person, i.e. balance or dis-ease. The first option, assumes that there is nothing wrong and the client or person just wants to improve their overall health and wellness. The second option, shows there is something that is wrong or some condition that needs to be addressed immediately and is out of balance.

These two options start right where we are at this moment in time. Option one, lets us know that the best time to focus on health and wellness is not when something is wrong, but when all is well and we want to just remain in good health, or improve our overall health and wellness. This is perfect since taking preventative measures will allow us to maintain our good health so we can continue to live well. The second option, assumes that we need to determine problems, and causes, and to provide solutions to bring about a condition of homeostasis, and then to improve and maintain our health and, balance and, to improve our living well in the future.

Change is the Beginning

Why change? The status quo is always apparent. If we want to do something different, we must apply change. For example, if we smoke cigarettes and want to stop smoking, we first must make up our mind to change. Second, we must agree to change on a permanent basis. This is not a temporary change such as not eating meat for a week. A permanent change will require commitment and an internal mental commitment, as well as physical change. Then we must apply the change and adapt to allow the change to take place. This is important, because the first phase will be to review the change we have implemented to see if we want to totally commit to it. Once the change is implemented, we can then make it a part of our daily routine. For example, if one sits on the coach and drinks beer everyday, but then decides to change and limit the couch sitting, activate an exercise routine and stop drinking beer, it will require much in the way of changing daily habits and routines to adjust to the new routine. If successful, one can change their lifestyle to a new one that will facilitate improving their health. So, as you can see, change is important. I had a friend that ate a lot of fried foods including a lot of meat and pork. It was affecting her health and weight. One day, after much discussion and contemplation, she decided to cut out the fried foods, stop eating pork and to limit her meat intake for more healthy vegetables. It was quite a commitment, because her friends and family ate a lot of fried foods and pork, but she decided to make the change in the best interest of her health and stuck to it.

Her commitment was a success, and it changed her eating habits and lifestyle. Change is not just a conversation about what I should or should not do and the pros and cons. Change is an action that takes place once a person decides or makes up their mind and puts it into action. I used to eat meat, then I decided to change and now I have been a vegetarian for 40 years. Change is an altering of one's behavior. Simple for some people, and not so simple for others. Some can make negative changes, affecting their health and some people can make positive changes to their behavior easily. Easy or difficult human behavior is affected by the changes we make in our lifestyle. The behavioral changes can make all the difference and are required if we want to improve our health and change habits, if necessary.

In Conclusion

So as we begin to make healthy changes in our life in order to heal and live well, it will require changes to be made, some minimal and some deeper, but we can do it if we put our minds to it and agree to accept changes that are for the betterment of our lives and wellbeing. If you think you can do it, you can. If you think you cannot, you won't. Commitment is required and is the brick in between the mortar because it will determine if we are really going to do something, or if we are just pontificating to our audience. It will determine how serious we are and if we are truthful to our own decision and level of commitment. Once we make the decision to change our current behavior or habit we must then implement the change.

How Does One Implement the Change Paradigm in their Life?

This is not a simple task for some people. Many people are not comfortable with change, even if it is for the better. One must implement this paradigm to change from unhealthy to healthy one day at a time. This begins with day one, by choosing to do an internal self scan, which will outline information that can be used to begin the journey to optimum health and living well. For instance, if I determine I need to make any changes in my life, I have to first sit down and determine where I am at this moment in time. We call this a baseline analysis. This will question and answer a group of parameters about my general health and expose more specific information. The next step is to address specific indications that are present or have presented themselves to show that I need to address certain situations or problems. Or, I just need to check to see if I am missing some hidden indicators beyond my own awareness and how to address these needs. Once my scan is completed, then I can address the specifics with my health counselor and create a prognosis of what I need to learn, understand, or do to change certain conditions, and how to determine if I am out of balance. This includes how to get back into a state of balance, good health, and wellness. This scan can be a blueprint, one I can use to keep myself in balance and in a state of good health. This blueprint will include a variety of physical and mental indicators that cover the total person. This is a holistic approach to help you to change your mind in order to implement change in your life.

Careful

One has to be very careful when making changes that can have an effect on their life and/or lifestyle. This is not simple, and many factors are to be weighed in the balance. For example, if you change the "A" factor, how does it affect the "B" factor. Like, if I become a vegetarian, how do I get enough protein or iron? If I decide to work two full time jobs, will I get enough sleep? Just a couple of examples, but changes do make a difference and so must be carefully considered. Also, what is the best approach for me to take has to be considered. I tried to help a person, but they did not consider they would never give up pork, which was affecting their health adversely. Dr. Atkins' original approach was to only eat meat, but later, he changed it to include a more balanced approach.

In Conclusion

Change has to be weighed to determine if it is gradual or too drastic to implement immediately. Questions need to be answered to determine if the change is holistic, so that the internal systems can absorb the changes without any detrimental side effects. One can change their behavior if they are committed to it, especially if it is for the betterment of self.

VII

The Holistic Approach

This is the beginning of seeking the whole person "wholistically." We begin with the physical approach, similar to a person getting a checkup from their Doctor on a yearly visit. This is similar, even if there is nothing done that is invasive. One can get a general checkup that just covers the basics to determine if you are in good general health, and if there is nothing you are complaining about. Secondly, the general checkup includes internal and observational analysis. That is where it stops, and there is a baseline of parameters that predetermine if one is in basic general health. If any of the parameters are out of predetermined limits, then further analysis is sometimes required. But it's not always done, because the Doctor prefers to wait several months to check again, especially if you are not complaining; this is unless the criteria sets off an alarm that requires immediate treatment, or your life is in imminent risk or danger. The difference with holistic medicine is that once the basic tests are complete, the Doctor or Health Counselor then checks the mental and metaphysical criteria to determine if there is more going on than what meets the eye. For example, if one is in good health, there may be mental issues that must be determined and explored to see if there are hidden things going on in the background, so to speak. Like if one is having pain or if a person is not breathing well, there may be some hidden stress or tension that is weakening their internal systems. This must be addressed, because the root cause of the weakening of their internal systems may be due to pent up anger, depression, hate, or worry, to name a few. Taking a painkiller might dull the senses for a time, but the underlying causal factors are still there; similar to a broken live electrical wire that an innocent person touches, then finds the wire is alive and dangerous to touch. There may be emotional things in their life that need to be addressed and mitigated before the person can heal, and become balanced, and restored to good health.

Holistic Medicine and healing requires more than a Band-Aid or a pill. It may require a much deeper analysis to get to the root cause of the problem or why a person is not in optimum health and wellness. As you know, many people do not like to discuss deeper issues of their personal lives with others and/or strangers and may not want to even talk to family or their Doctor. So it requires some tact, and a deeper understanding of the total person on a mental, physical and spiritual level. The average doctor is trained to focus on the exposed physical symptom(s). For anything else, they will refer you to a specialist that may or may not focus on you totally or may just make a judgment call as to your specific physical problem. They may assume that the problem is real or all in your mind and prescribe some type of medicine (pill) to obscure the main or secondary problem that may be the cause. Since the cause is not addressed, the problem(s) never go away or may make way for new problems; or, you are given some medicine that will create a totally new problem or set of circumstances that will require more treatments for the side effects of the pills. This is why holistic medicine is of value in determining the cause of problems, and to provide solutions that will heal the existing problem (cause), not create new ones, and will balance the person back to health and a state of wellness.

Accepting Change

Acceptance is needed to make us move to the next step and begin to institute the changes we need to make our quest for better health, healing and wellness. For example, I helped a lady who had very bad arthritis and was in severe pain. Her hands were swollen, and she did not know what to do. The doctors could not help her, so she asked for my advice. My advice was to change her diet and not to eat pork, limit meats and eat vegetables and lots of citrus fruits. She agreed to the changes and accepted my advice. Within 3 months, her hands stopped hurting and the swelling in her hands subsided. Her health improved, and she was happy. Eight more months passed and I got a call that her problems and pain had returned. I questioned her, and she explained that she had gone back to her old habit of eating lots of pork and meats. I explained that she needed to stop eating pork, and she stated that she did not want to change because she loved pork and would rather suffer the pain and immobility of her hands than to give up pork. I understood that, and we said our goodbyes. Her daughter asked what I could do, but I explained that her mother refused to change and was content in her distress. She refused to change. In another case, I tried to convince a friend to stop smoking cigarettes; he refused, even though it was affecting his health. He suffered a health crisis but continued to smoke. I did not try to force him, as it is up to the individual to change; one has to want to.

In Conclusion

Holistically, we can help ourselves before we have a health crisis by changing what is adversely affecting us; by changing what is creating the problem. It may require us to change something in our lifestyle, but it is for the better. The holistic doctor will try and provide insight and information, so one can make educated decisions and change what is required for the betterment of the individual to improve their health and increase their wellbeing. So, change is important, and one must change their mind first, commit to the changes, and then implement the changes; lastly, they must maintain the changes once implemented after receiving positive results. You make the ultimate decisions and reap the benefits of the positive changes you make. These changes can be on different levels, but they are to help you heal or increase your wellbeing. So you must ask yourself what you need or what you need to address when it comes to your health.

I Met the Holistic Doctor

My only mistake
Is taking life for granted
Unsealed the information speaks
As my mind says hello to my heart
I feel easy and uneasy
As I reflect on what to do next
Stand up or sit down
Walk the walk
Talk but who is listening
I ponder the questions
I need to ask myself
And others
Am I all right?
Are we all right?
Do we need to take this and that?
To be alright
Is it in the food or the water
Is it in the air?
As I breathe in and out
The toxins of the day
Waiting for a break in the flow
I take a pill knowing it is not a panacea
But I hope the doctor is right and I am wrong
Or I am right to not take this pill
then the doctor is wrong
But intervention is near
Or, is it far as the water that flows away from me
To somewhere else is the antidote
Of my life as the tide ebbs and flows
For another day
In a another way
And brings in good news of the wane of new trials or tricks
That promise me the old side effects are over
As new ones come with a promise
That I am saved

I can live another day without the pain
Of not knowing what is going on
Until I reach out to see
A holistic doctor waiting to reveal news to me
Of a way to save myself from the disdain of new dis-eases
Side effects from the breeze
Of new scientific approaches
To the old cures that work
and nothing outside or ordinary
Is going to affect me
They have answered my question and holistically
Set me free and I am renewed
By the ancestors who bought me here
To live well and live pain and dis-ease free.

VIII

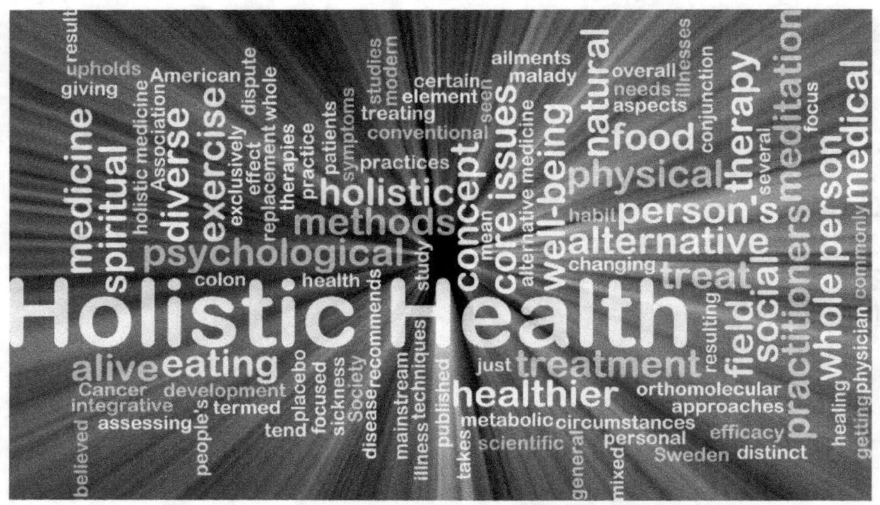

Health Question

The Query

Are you healthy? This is a question you can answer. It is either yes or no. If it is a maybe, then you need to get a basic checkup. If it is a yes, great, then you can ask the question, do you need to improve? If this is also a yes, then you can start with the basic and then an in-depth checkup to see how your health is. The first focus is to determine how healthy and balanced we are. Good, bad, excellent or needs improvement are the choices. All of us fall into one of these categories. It doesn't matter which, it just gives a starting point or place to begin the journey. If there is nothing to address in our health scan, great. If there is something or things we need to address, we now have a starting place and can move forward and determine the next step(s). Do you need to be healed? Are you healed partially or totally? Do you know what that means? It means that some are healed partially, but the problem keeps coming back. Totally healed means we are balanced and ok. Or do you need to heal? Are you living well?

The First Step

The first step is to perform a basic checkup of the physical system. This is normal and could be equivalent to the basic general checkup that one receives at any Doctor's office, whether it is performed by a general medical practitioner or a holistic medical practitioner. This checkup is required to check basic vitals to detect if all basic systems are normal. The vitals can check blood, breath, circulation, hormones, tongue and pulse analysis, visual observation, body structure, weight and anything that stands out as abnormal or triggers deeper analysis. This will provide a body of information to determine basically where a person is and will establish a baseline. Then, this information is evaluated for imbalances.

The Second Step

The second vital step is to fill out a questionnaire that is created by the holistic practitioner. The client, to provide obscure information previously unknown to the medical practitioner, must fill out this form. It is required because a deeper analysis is necessary to understand the total person. The questions will reveal information that will provide insight into what is not apparent from the basic checkup, such as what is happening on a mental or emotional or unknown level. This will give the client an opportunity to articulate anything that is bothering them or express what they think or know is going on with their health as they see it. It also can give them an opportunity to express important information that is needed by the holistic medical practitioner to make an educated prognosis. Something as simple as bowel movements or events happening in the client's life can impact their health and will not be picked up by a basic checkup. Also, has something happened with the family, or with work or their spouse or child? These are questions that can uncover information that can help the medical practitioner and the client to provide healing or insight into what is causing their health situation or causing an out-of-balance condition. For example, I met a woman who had multiple problems with her health. She was on several medications for high blood pressure and diabetes, to name a few, and her health was getting worse. I questioned her, had her fill out a questionnaire and learned that she was divorced; she divulged that she hated her husband to the nth degree. When I questioned her about when she last saw her husband, she stated that she had not seen or heard from him for eight years. I then realized that the prognosis was her hate for him, and that needed to change. It was so great that she was creating an out-of-balance condition that seriously affected her health. My prescription was to go home and redecorate her bedroom, to begin to take long walks, and to exhale all the hate she harbored for her ex-husband out of her internal system, including her mind and heart, and then return in three months for a follow up. After six months, her health had improved so that her high blood pressure and diabetes were disappearing. She realized that she was now healing and her health was improving, and she was now coming into balance. Her health had been affected by her emotions and her negative mental attitude. She changed her mind, her thinking, and her heart, and her health changed at the same time.

The Third Step

The third step is to now to perform the oral exam, which is vital and required. Once the first two steps are completed, then step three is to sit down and go over the information collected and to confirm that there is some basic consensus, and then go deeper and ask any outstanding questions, confirm a diagnosis, and determine if there is anything missing or needed to confirm the overall analysis and the resultant prognosis. All of the findings are discussed, and anything else that needs to be revealed or expressed is accomplished in this step. Any agreements or disagreements are discussed and confirmed or nullified. It is then time to discuss cause(s) and solution(s) and any further analyses required. Any prescriptions are then discussed and affirmed and a follow up is scheduled if required.

In Conclusion

So, as we learn that we must consider the whole person in our quest to help our clients, we must analyze the total person, not just basic vital physical statistics. There is more than just physical vital statistics that need to be determined and analyzed. We must interview and include the total person. Also, realize that mental and emotional upsets can cause physical problems. At the same time, changing our minds can affect our health in a positive way. This is why it is important to talk with the client or patient and try to understand the whole person, and what is affecting them on other than purely physical levels. Asking questions helps to get answers, which can reveal causal data that will lead to effective solutions for the client. It will also help you to make a better-informed diagnosis and create a better prognosis for your client.

IX

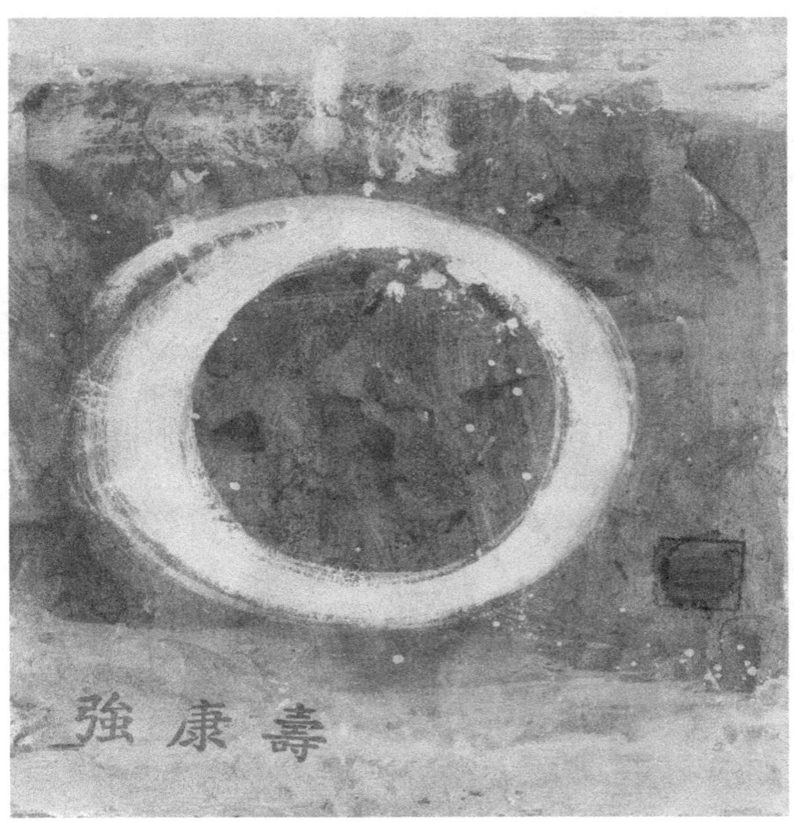

The Dao

The Journey

The first step is enacting change protocols. Begin the journey from where you are to where you need to be. If you are out of balance, then it is time to begin to become balanced. If you are not whole, then it is time to be whole. If you are diseased, it is time to become well.

If you are not in the best of health, it is time to improve your health. It is a step-by-step, day-by-day process. For example, if I am stiff, it is time to become more flexible. How, you say? First, I must begin to do some exercises such as stretching, yoga or different physical movements that help my joints and muscles to loosen up and twist. If I am weak, then I must begin to do exercises that help to strengthen my body. Now, you may think becoming flexible is easy, but it is not. I must also become flexible in my mind at the same time, so I am stretching not only my body, but also my mind. If one hates or has a grudge against someone, then it is time to let go of that grudge or that hate from the heart and replace love in the inner and mental space. This is why they say, "Let it go." Let go of the old limiting mindset so that one can become flexible, more open and have the ability to extend their mental capacity.

What to Let Go of From Your Heart/Mind

Worry
Tension
Anxiety
Stress
Fear
Hate
Negativity
Grudges
Lack of confidence
Wrong beliefs
Old stuff (past)
Issues that do not help you

Dis-ease
Nonsense
Mistakes past and present
Illusions
Lies
Doubt that you cannot change or improve

As we start to put in place the changes necessary to progress and change what is required, we have to see and experience some proof that what we are doing is actually working. For example, people take pills for headaches year one and, year ten, still have the headaches, which means that the pills did not work. Working temporarily does not mean it worked. When the headaches subside and do not return, it means it worked. This is the test that we have to utilize to prove we are on the right road and the changes we are enacting are indeed working. Now, do not expect it to work immediately, unless it does. I have seen changes work immediately and I have seen changes that work over a certain amount of time. In the latter case, it required some amount of time for the changes to take hold and show progress or success. If one wants to lose weight, it takes time to lose weight (just as it took time to gain), but as one works toward their target goal they will see and feel some small achievement, such as their weight becomes less or their waistline reduces or they can now fit into those jeans that previously they could not. We may have to tweak our changes so that they are more effective, and we must add or subtract anything that is needed or is not working. I once had a client who could not gain weight; she was on thyroid medicine, but it did not help. After querying her and asking the right questions, I discovered a little-known fact. This lady liked to do two and a half hours of high step aerobics, which was burning off any weight gains. I explained to her to only do an hour to one hour and a half, and so she changed her routine. One year later, she had gained the weight, reaching her goal. The Doctor who prescribed her thyroid medicine did not enquire about the activities in her daily life.

As we implement those things or steps we need to take in order to change our lives or behavior, it takes perseverance and commitment. This means staying the course and just continuing on the path to success. If we are to improve our circulation, we have to exercise or walk or jog until we make small improvements and eventually larger improvements. We have to remember the mind can change in an instant, but the body needs some finite amount of time to enact our changes and show marked improvement until success and permanent change.

In Conclusion

We can change, we can improve, and we can succeed. It may be in an instant to change our mind but need more time to improve, enact changes and make the necessary changes permanent. Let me give you an example. I used to eat meat, chicken and fish. One day, I decided to stop eating meat for one week. At the end of the week I succeeded in keeping to my decision and did not eat any meat. At the end of the week, I celebrated and then made a more permanent decision to not eat any more meat and become a vegetarian. I removed all flesh of any kind from my diet and my home and began my journey to become a vegetarian. Each day I saw meat and resisted any temptation to eat meat or chicken or fish; more than thirty-five years later, I am still a vegetarian. I was able to change my mind, change my habit, stick to my decision, stick to it, and persevere. I succeeded and reached my goal.

This is similar to how we reach and attain all kinds of goals, mini and major, and it works the same way for the goal of optimum health and wellness. As you reach stages of improvement in your health and wellness, any problems that come up must be addressed. Your steps and changes must be critiqued; any tweaking can be made, and what is working or not working can be addressed. This appears to be scientific, but it is not. It is applied, and so as we make necessary changes, we can get some immediate or delayed feedback.

Feedback

The most important thing when making changes is feedback. If I make changes, I must see that they are working and get feedback that the changes work or do not work or need some tweaking. Once I realize the changes are working and are good changes, I can continue the journey toward my goal. If the changes you make are working, stick to them. If the changes are not working, then let's determine what is not correct or what is not working. For example, once, some ladies wanted to be healthy because they were experiencing some disease. They were put on a regimen and were told that they must stick to it for six months to a year without deviation. There were two major requirements that must be met. They were no smoking and no alcohol. They all agreed to the requirements. They were given some herbs and a proper diet and were sent home to make the necessary changes. There were six ladies, and after six months they were queried to see their progress. Four of the ladies did well and were on their way to remarkable improvements in their health. Two ladies did not show an improvement. They also lied about sticking to the two requirements that were imperative, no smoking and no alcohol. But they thought they were smarter than anyone else. We knew they were not telling the truth, and after much querying they admitted that they were smoking and drinking alcohol. They did not succeed and left the program, because they had not improved and, subsequently, there was no improvement in their health. So, commitment to yourself and to the changes and goal(s) you would like to achieve is important. Commitment to the goals and the need to stick to the journey is how we get there, so we can attain our goals. This does require some inner strength and willpower.

Inner Strength and Willpower

As one knows, one cannot get anywhere without instituting inner strength to stick to the course to reach their ultimate goal(s). It is easy to say one can and will do, but to actually do what one says is quite another; it is an accomplishment to be strong enough to complete the task(s) before them. Inner strength is coupled with willpower. Willpower is the gift we have to accomplish much that we do and to help us with our decision-making abilities in order to make certain decisions, such as to smoke cigarettes or not to, or to use drugs, quit using drugs or not to use drugs at all. Many times, it is our willpower we use to make better choices for ourselves, as opposed to choices that other people like to make for us that are not for our best or highest good. The will to succeed is pushing us to complete our goals. So, in order to stick to what we set out to do or accomplish, our willpower helps us on our journey. For some, this is enough, but for others whose belief systems are challenged or not strong enough, we need to incorporate faith in our own selves and abilities.

Faith

We live and move by faith. The faith that we can, and can do, and can attain our goals. It you do not believe, then it will not happen. If you do not have faith in yourself, then you will not do what is required wholeheartedly and will possibly not start, or will sabotage or quit before reaching your goals, which may be right around the turn. **Believe** in yourself, have faith you can and you will succeed, and try and make the necessary steps. All journeys begin with the first step. Do not let people convince you that you cannot do or accomplish. Or, the other point is they will make you feel you are weak (willpower) and you will doubt yourself.

In Conclusion

Willpower is required to make changes and to stick to those decisions. Even if we believe we must trust our self to have the confidence and use our willpower go through with it and stay with it until we reach our goal. You can affirm that you have strong willpower everyday or write it on a note and post it on the mirror until we feel it is no longer necessary as our willpower improves. Remember believe in your self.

X

Understanding the Total Person: Body, Mind, Spirit

Awareness is not only for observing the physical. It is for one to begin to understand the complexity of who you are. The total person is the physical body, the mind and the Spirit. This is the "Wholistic" view, which one endeavors to learn, and understand. This is the level of awareness one must know and is also the total person health and/or
medical practitioners must understand. This "Wholistic" approach must be brought to bear when trying to heal a person or maintain the health and wealth of any individual we are assisting as a client. You must see yourself as multidimensional, and the health and medical practitioners must see you the same way, since men and women are not one-dimensional.

The totality of a person is to be considered when helping them to be and remain balanced in a state of homeostasis. The sage or the medical practitioner must see you, and all you bring with you, to understand the root cause of any problems or health issues you may have. The problem can be physical or it can just be mental or emotional, which may be temporary in nature and can be dismissed once addressed and a solution applied to correct the problem. One such condition can cause a person to be out of balance, which may have a negative effect upon the person's health due to an emotional problem, such as a divorce or loss of a love one or severe financial difficulty. There is no external physical cut to apply a Band-Aid to, but it will require Band-Aids that are of an invisible mental nature to correct the physical outbreak of dis-ease(s) so the person can get back to balance and ease. So, the nature of traditional and natural medicine, deemed alternative, always takes or should take into account the total person regarding their body, mind and Spirit before applying the remedy to remove the cause and consummate the solution. This is to ensure that the person does not come back again with the same reoccurring problem, because it was not healed correctly due to a lack of exposing the root cause. This happens by only looking at the physical expression, which might be just the alarm or smoke and not the fire.

There is a reason why there are two sides to a coin, and people are more than two sides of the same coin. We are all multidimensional inside and out.

Internal Versus External

You have an external and an internal part, and both work together to keep you healthy. Without the inner, there is no outer, and vice versa. So, we should know and understand both, not just what is viewed in the mirror. The external is for all to see. The internal is for you to know and understand. Both have to be maintained by you and, when maintained well, one has good health and will feel wealthy. Many rewards come with that, including long life and the ability to live well. Internal includes vital organs, blood, energy, hormones, fluids and nerves. External includes the core, the limbs, the eyes, the skin, the head and the feet. So, we have to include all that is within and all that is without. All is included that we can see as well as all that we cannot see, including our mind and thoughts.

Mind and Matter

The mind or mental attitude is a part of the whole person. So, what does that mean? Can we think what we want? Can we think negatively or positively? Does it make a difference? So, does a good mental attitude help? Belief systems are a part of our mind or mental attitude. Yes, we can think what we want. We cannot do all we want, as there are some limits imposed, but it does not stop us from thinking good or bad. What do you think, about you or others? Do good thoughts or bad thoughts matter to you?

Thoughts are Things

What are you thinking about? Are you thinking about your health or your money? Are you thinking negative thoughts or positive thoughts, or are you thinking about healing thoughts? What you think can affect your health in a positive or negative way. Do you think you are sick or well? Do you love yourself or hate yourself? Do you send yourself negative thoughts or positive thoughts? Are you thinking less of yourself, as opposed to thinking that you are ok and being the best? Do you exaggerate when you have a minor problem, such as a cold? Do you think that you are gravely ill or think you are ok and will get better very soon? So, what is on your mind about you? Think good thoughts instead of bad thoughts, especially when thinking about yourself. Are you loving yourself for you, and not thinking the worst about how you look or your hair or how tall or short or thin or fat? Think you are ok, no matter what the circumstance. Thoughts are also things, and those things can affect your health and wellbeing. Are you your own best friend, or do you hate the person you are? Love yourself and stop thinking less of yourself; think you are perfect the way you are, especially today, when many want to change body parts and create anything other than who they are. Or, they hate who they are and how they look in the mirror. When you are not feeling well, instead of thinking the worst, think you are healing, ok, and getting well. Thinking positive creates positive things. Instead of thinking sick thoughts, think you are healing or healed.

In Conclusion

Thinking is not doing, so thinking is great, but one must also do and not just think about doing. Turn those positive thoughts into doing positive things. If you want to make yourself better, think better thoughts. No surgeon is going to make you a better person. You are more than just a physical body, and you need to use your gifts of inner strength, willpower and faith and believe in you, not some TV character that is being paid to act a certain way with a script. This is the true reality.

XI

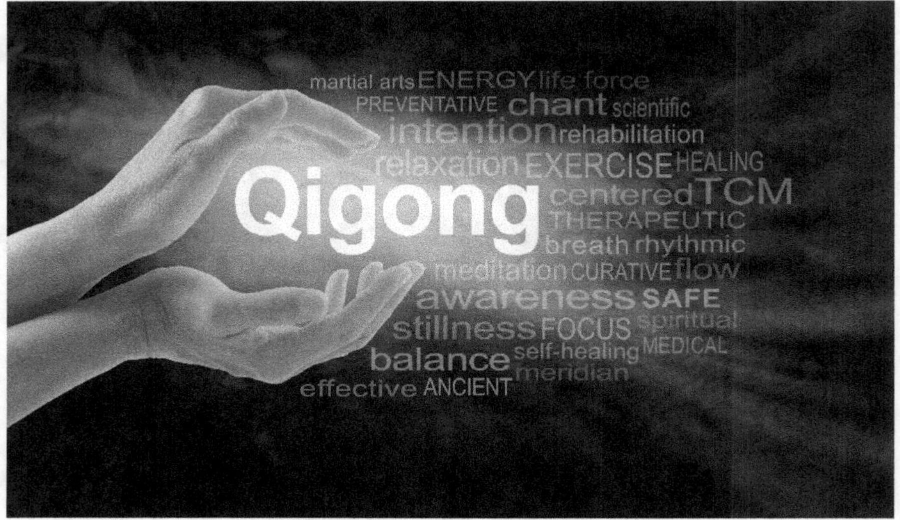

Qigong Healing

Healing

When you have a problem, such as you notice you are hot or you are cold, do you think first a thought of healing? Do you think you can heal? Do you think you can heal yourself? Will healing thoughts help you? Yes, healing thoughts can help you, and it can also help you to have a healing state of mind. What it takes to heal can be simple or can be complex, but you first want to place your mind in a "healing state of mind." What will it take to heal yourself is a great question; second to, what will it take to heal? This can be done with proper assistance from medical or alternative health professionals. The truth is that medical professionals can only help you to heal, or your body to heal itself. So, the first and most important step is to think I can heal; I can and I will heal. 'I am healed' is thinking a thought, tantamount to using a thought to create a thing or positive outcome, which is, "I am healed."

Requirements for Healing

Believe
State of mind
Finding the cause
Provide a solution(s)
Action (change in lifestyle)
Trust
Patience
Corrective measures
State of mind
Affirmation: "I am healed"
Spiritual and mental understanding
Healing complete confirmation
Maintain changes and balance
Learned lesson

What you think and believe is very important and will help you heal any problem that you may have. Your state of mind always comes into play, since if we are in a positive frame of mind we think positive thoughts, and as we know, thoughts are things. Once we believe and are in a positive state of mind, conducive to healing, we can look for or discover the cause of our problem. Finding the cause of any problem is tantamount to finding the solution. Even though we believe, we must trust that we can heal after finding the cause and implementing the proper solution. At that point, we have to then trust our self and be patient enough for the solution to take place and be open to any corrections that may need to be added to ensure success. Again, we continue to remember to keep a positive state of mind, and affirm that we are healing and will be healed. This will then require that we evaluate what we have learned or are learning from the problem and the eventual solution to be fully healed. There may be a lesson learned so that the problem or circumstance does not repeat itself again. After we are fully healed, we should confirm to ourselves that we are fully healed and not doubt ourselves, and then stick to any required changes we have to make in our current lifestyle to maintain a level of optimum health, balance and wellbeing.

Sometimes, we cannot heal because we do not understand what is happening or the lesson we are learning or should have learned. Healing also requires us to appreciate the Higher Source of our ability and the gift of healing. We also should not spend time blaming everyone else or ourselves for what has transpired; instead, we should focus on the present moment and the healing. This why we see many people, no matter their beliefs, pray for healing and help when they are afflicted or not well. They pray for the Higher Source to assist or heal them and to bring them back into a state of balance and health. This includes what is happening in the universe and what is happening in our daily lives. This includes what we think and what we do to ourselves, including what we ingest into our bodies. Does eating unhealthy food make us healthy? Does thinking unhealthy thoughts make us healthy? Everything we do or do not do has an effect, whether it is minor or major.

Is Food Our Foe or Friend

To eat meat or to be vegetarian; is there a choice? What is the question? Is junk food good and healthy, or just good? Will food make us healthy or not? Is herbal the way? Is good nutrition important, or just not true? Does putting chemicals into soil and on the food being grown have an adverse affect on our health and us? It has been studied for years, and the empirical analysis proves it does have an effect; just giving hormones to animals can cause a problem with humans that ingest the meat. Some say that violently killing animals causes the secretion of hormonal chemicals that are not good for human beings. The mind can affect hormones, and so can food. Many choose to eat organic, and it is proving that it can help control the amount of harmful chemicals we ingest and strike a balance within our internal system, which fosters good health.

Balance

Balance: what does it mean? The definition of balance states that it is an even distribution of weight enabling someone or something to remain upright and steady. In health, it is the balance that allows a person to be in good health within and without. In our life, we understand the balance of work versus play or the balance of nutritious food versus junk food or being awake versus getting proper rest, or the supposed balance between the scales of justice. So, since we are familiar with what balance is, we have to understand that our life is lived in the balance of what is and what it is supposed to be.

Balance is everywhere in the land of opposites. Ponder these below.

Earth universe
Awake sleep
Work play
Quiet noisy
See blind
TV music
Sit move
Run walk
Nutritious food junk food
Cooked food raw food
Water wine/whiskey
Juice tea
Peace war
Calm angry
Sad happy
Love hate
Relationship alone
Justice crime
Clean dirty

Rich poor
Well sick
Intelligent illiterate
Clear cloudy
Laugh cry
Eat starve
Care don't care
Friend enemy
Right wrong
Health wealth

Do we consider these when we think of balance in our lives, or do we not see the balance we juggle on a daily basis? Consequently, we must apply that balance within our health and must maintain our health and ensure that we keep it in balance. For example, our blood pressure has a balance between sodium and potassium within the body. There is a balance between good HDL and bad LDL. We have many balances between normal and abnormal hormonal levels within our body. Our weight also has a balance; that is how we determine who is at weight or overweight or underweight, even if it is subjective. So, we should strive to maintain balance within our bodies and our life's activities. Also, we should know that one important balance is the energy, within our body.

Our Energy of Life

Our body has yin (negative energy) and yang (positive) energy, and the balance is different for men and women, but we both have the same energy, just in a difference balance quotient. For example, men have a lot of yang energy, and a small amount of yin energy to balance their energy system. Women have a lot of yin energy, and a small amount of yang energy in their energetic system. The Chinese culture has a yin/yang system to illustrate the balance of internal energy. When these energetic systems go out of balance, then a person will feel out of balance energetically. It is relativity easy to get back to balance and rebalance your energetic system.

Energy is everywhere in the Universe, so we do not have to worry that there is a shortage in the Universe, but we have to maintain and ensure we have enough energy within our bodies. So, again, we have to balance our energetic systems to not use up all of our internal energy. This includes the energy we are born with, gifted to us from our parents, and the food we eat to replenish our energy by eating nutritious foods and herbs. If we are able to maintain good energy levels, we will feel strong and in balance as we go through our day full of numerous activities. As we rest, we replenish and balance our energetic systems. This goes a long way to how we feel and participate in life and assists us in moving from surviving to living well.

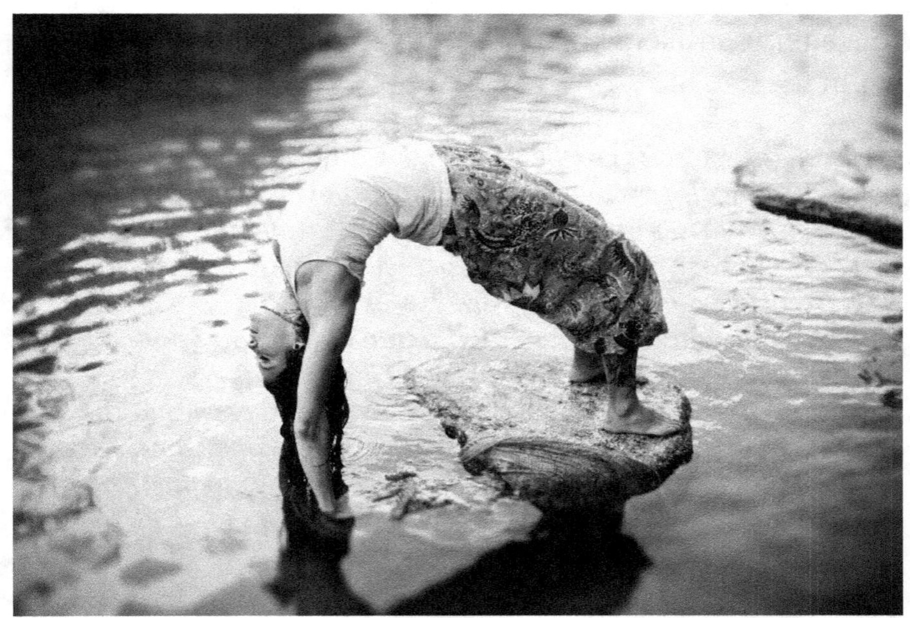

Yoga Practice

Exercise for Healing

Exercise for healing or as a medicine can help cure maladies if the assigned or prescribed exercises are taken seriously and completed over time at the rate required to improve and change whatever the dis- ease is. This idea that exercise is medicine is not new. Many traditional cultures used exercise as a way to heal maladies that could not be healed without invasive interventions. Exercise as medicine can be safely designed, prescribed and if completed can correct serious out of balance condition that otherwise would be treated with some type of drug(s). For example, to decrease obesity, one must use exercise as a modality and practice certain types of exercises that can burn calories and strengthen the overall system by increasing muscle strength. This excerpt explains this point:

*"Prescribing exercise can be an effective alternative to traditional pharmaceuticals for conditions that are known to respond to exercise. While it is often thought that increasing physical activity will only improve health markers associated with obesity (hypertension, diabetes, heart disease, etc.), in **2015, the Scandinavian Journal of Medicine and Science in Sports** highlighted the use of exercise as medicine to treat 26 chronic conditions and showed using evidence based research that the use of physical activity is effective in treating these conditions. However, despite the strong evidence for exercise, helping patients change their physical activity behaviors continues to be a challenge for healthcare providers."*

In Conclusion

Exercise can improve and heal all types of non-communicable diseases such as cardiovascular diseases, degenerative diseases, muscular atrophy diseases, respiratory diseases, diabetes, osteoarthritis, hypertension, and brain related diseases, to name a few. In China, for example, exercise as medicine is prevalent everywhere in their society because they realize:

- The cost of medicine is too expensive, especially if you do not have insurance.
- Surgery and invasive approaches do not provide a panacea of remedies
- Pharmaceutical approaches may not be effective because of side effects that are inherent in the drugs
- Exercise has very small or no side effects and is a passive way to achieve the goal

● Exercise can heal and promote longevity

Exercises one can do in addition to their regular daily activity, will improve your flexibility, strength, coordination, or endurance. Exercise can be completed lying in bed, sitting, standing, through movement, such as walking, running or riding a bike, and in the water, such as aerobics. This can help you attain goals in health and fitness, and help one to live well, and live longer. At the same time, exercise can and will increase mental stimulation and improve brain function.

XII

From Surviving to Living Well

Are we surviving, or are we living well? Do we know the difference? Is life about surviving, or it is about living well? Many people want to live well and, as a child, you think you are here to live well; if your parents are surviving, you think that when you become an adult, you will change the paradigm and live well. This is only to find out that you do not understand life as you know it, because for most, your parents do not tell you the "real deal" or reality because they want you to remain positive, hopeful, and untainted from the cons of daily life. They expound on the pros of life, and try to guide you into adulthood with the idea that it is there for the taking (life). You, as a young adult, then step into the reality of life, and it is different for each person, especially if you are born with a gold or silver spoon, or you have to work for all that you get or achieve and you literally have to save yourself and, if you are lucky, you and your family. Some are thrust into life at a very early age for whatever reason and have to hit the ground running, then spend most of their life trying to survive. Surviving means having a roof over your head, food in your belly or for the family, and clothes on your back. This includes some modest furniture, a modest car and some basic amenities like a TV, computer and smart phone. This might seem very basic, but some do not have that. Some have to work two jobs to do this. No time to look after their health. The biggest dilemma is how you take care of your health, because that is paramount, everything else considered. Some people immediately begin surviving like a swimmer treading water as bills come fast and frequent and so does the growth of the family, which then places pressure to make sure everyone is ok, just ok. So many focus on feeding the family and putting enough food on the table and not about the quality of the food. Choices are made with the idea of surviving and not about what one prefers or the idea of living well.

I discovered in poorer neighborhoods many people were focused on survival and not on living well, because most of their income was to support only basics; the idea of living well was a dream deferred, but hopeful. This dilemma was real, and many did surviving well. They met the basic requirements outlined earlier of food on the table, a roof over their heads and clothes on their back. The cost in their neighborhoods was expensive, but getting the most "bang" for your dollar was not realized. Nobody discussed nutrition, they confirmed "belly full." When you are focused on surviving, the idea of living well does not come into play. You work, make money and pay bills, with no rest for the weary. Many times, it offers no balance in lifestyle. It is take care of the basic staples, and life is good. When you enquire about the concept of living well, many people state that surviving is good and living well is a concept that comes with a hefty price tag or is not in their present neighborhood. This is far from the truth. One of the main criteria of living well is the idea of being healthy and living a balanced life for the entire family. Even if one is alone, one should live well also.

The idea of living well is based on choices that one has the ability to make each and every day in their life. It is not based on survival, which focuses on little or no individual choices. For example, I want to live an organic, vegetarian lifestyle with a balance between work, exercise and play, with plenty of vacations that allow me to travel the world. I intend to eat proper, nutritious, organic foods that are not GMO engineered, but organically grown with love and patience as the only fertilizer and insecticide. I like clothes that are of high quality materials that are also chemically free and in a house that is modern, with all the amenities and VCO painted walls, bamboo flooring and air purification systems, climate controls room by room, with a salt water pool out back. Sounds nice, but comes with a price tag that encumbers my possibility of living well. Is all of this is needed? Is living well out of reach?

No, living well can be obtained exactly where I am in my small apartment or house, but I choose to spend my little money on what my choices demand, such as organic and nutritious foods. This is easy to do, even if I have to grow it in the backyard or on the fire escape. I can take mini vacations and can spend evenings after dinner on walks to relax and breathe the aroma of fresh air. I can choose to buy clothes that are of a nice quality instead of focusing on quantity. I can paint my home with VCO paint and ensure there is no lead paint, and keep the air clean with air filters and an air purifier if I need one. I can take time to exercise, even if it is only a very short period each and every day or a few times a week. I can choose to cut back on chemicals, high fructose sugars and the extensive salts that are added to prepared foods. I can choose to cook instead of living the microwave style of TV dinners. I can cook at home instead of eating out at the fast food drive thru that dot or impale the local environment. I can limit the foods that are not nutritional for myself and the family instead of just focusing on the idea of just filling their bellies. I can do things or activities that make one feel satisfied or happy that are not focused on just something you have to do, like a chore such as putting out the trash. So, the secret to living well is available to all, but requires one to make choices that fulfill needs and wants and is not solely focused on cost or the cheapest cost, but this is best for me and/or my family.

Quality Versus Quantity

Choices have to do many times with quantity versus quality. Necessity versus wants, such as I want food that is cheap or I want non-GMO foodstuffs or regular food versus organic foods. I can have twenty cheap tee shirts that shrink or ten quality cotton tee shirts that look and feel new after they are washed. Choices determine quality versus quantity. Our decision-making determines what is best, or what is so-so or barely satisfies what we determine is acceptable without forgoing our own criteria of what is or what one can get by with. Many times, we think it is only price that is the choice, but this is not true. The decision is on us to set our own criteria and to then fulfill them based on our own standards that will help us to fulfill our desire to live healthy and live well.

Living Well: What is That?

Is that different than just living, or "I am ok"? We all think that we are living ok; some think they are living better than others, since they may have more things or more money, or their home and living conditions are better. Or, our local environment is better or best, like living in a million-dollar neighborhood in your million-dollar house. Although, there are some who have very little and think they are ok even though they have the minimum, but they are happy and are satisfied with what they do have. Then, there are those who have nothing and think they are living well, even if they are begging for what they need and have no home, but no everyday pressures to pay insurmountable bills and responsibilities that some have to deal with on a daily basis. So, you see, it is all relative to how and what you think makes you ok, satisfied and possibly living well; if not, you are still "ok."

You ask, aren't we all living well? The answer we wish would be yes, but actually, it is no. Part of the reason is because many people do not know what it is to live well and how to live well. It is not a course they teach in college or continuing education. It is more of an on-the-job, self-taught curriculum that we are forced to learn while doing the best or worse we can, or somewhere in between. For example, we live in a neighborhood we do not like, in a house we do not want to live in, with people we wish would move or allow you to move, and every day when you go home, you dread it, but deal with it in hopes that it and the circumstances will change.

Or, do you consider living well eating lobster and abalones, pizza, burgers, KFC chicken and mountains of sweets, or do you feel living well is nutritious, somewhat bland foodstuffs? It is all relative to what you think and consider is your idea of living well. When I asked a friend what he considered living well, he stated it was sitting on the front porch in a rocking chair. I asked another person, and he stated it was going to an all-inclusive resort with a drink in his hand 24/7. Another young guy told me it was not working and just watching sports on TV. Another young lady told me she only wanted to do yoga and ballroom dancing all day, and that is all. So, we all have some idea as to living well, whether we are doing it or not. Some are living well according to their own definition and others are living their dream, and then there are many who want to know what "living well" looks like so they can start doing it instead of it being a hope or a dream deferred by necessity. Everyone deserves to live well, and it should be a minimum requirement for all. So, let's explore more about living well.

How Does One Live Well?

How does one live well? Does one spend the most money, and now they are living well, or is it the biggest house and the most toys to play with or eating the richest foods? In the Babylon online dictionary, the definition of living well is to "live in luxury, live free of financial worries." Is this it, or is there something else? In China, the idea of living well is to have enough to eat, a place to rest, proper clothes and a good family, and that you exercise every day and have good health. In America, living well is having money and luxuries; health does not come high on the list. Some people think that you can buy health or, as some will say, the best doctors are at your disposal. Having the best doctors at your disposal does not mean you have good health or can be healed. It means you are putting health first so that you will not need those expensive doctors.

 Many traditional cultures in so-called third world countries place health before wealth, because one can get sick and lose their wealth paying for the expensive doctors. So, the consensus is that living well does include wealth, but should not be before health. In a country that is supposed to be so rich, you would think someone in government is wise enough to place health and welfare above all for its citizens, but that does not happen in the world's "richest country." This is due to the fact that healthcare in America is a business, not a service provided for its citizens. There needs to be a paradigm shift in thinking to provide healthcare for all in the USA, whether one can afford it or not.

So, this requires one to provide their own healthcare and wellbeing. One has to learn to live well no matter the circumstances, and not rely on the government to provide things, by focusing on health and what it takes to be and remain healthy and to learn how to live well from a young age to an ancient age. Hopefully, we all agree that we are responsible for our own health and to live well (wellbeing).

Do You Know How to Live Well?

Living well requires several steps that everyone can take and complete to try and live the best life, one that includes optimum health and wellbeing. First, one must look to their health to see where they are. Then, one must look at their life and determine where they are at the same time. This is similar to an overall evaluation that focuses on the present moment. This is to determine where you are and what is positive or negative; what the needs and wants are, and how one is doing presently. One must check the health and see what requires improvement or what changes need to be made. This includes what needs to be healed and bought into balance. Then, one must discuss what will make them feel that they are living well and what is missing, and how to provide the missing link or ingredients. Once that is completed, then it will be time to implement a plan to achieve the goals that are agreed upon through the evaluation process. Once everyone understands what it takes to live well, then action is taken to accomplish this over a period of time and then to maintain this wellbeing going forward. Living well may be different for each person, but it still can be achieved, especially when it comes to general health. If you do not know the difference below is a listed of clues to tell if you are just surviving. In the next chapter there is another list that outlines some of the aspects of living well that can be used as a basic guide to understanding what wellbeing or living well is to you as an individual.

How to Tell You Are Just Surviving

Just making ends meet and satisfied with that
Focusing on quantity, not on quality
On welfare, but have a brilliant mind and college degree
Focusing on what you can get cheaply, not what is good for your health or your children's health
Willing to live in squalor instead of cleaning up; blaming it on our life as a child
Will not buy organic because you don't get a large quantity
Do the minimum to get by
Suffering, but refuse to make changes to stop the suffering
Depressed at current situation and does nothing to change it
Thinking and worrying, but <u>doing nothing about it</u>
Won't make a decision to change what is causing you pain
Will not take advice that will help you
Waiting for success to come grab you off the couch
Rather beg than work for what you need

Won't love yourself
You hate yourself
Rather be homeless
Hiding from self and others
Can do better but scare
Living with fear in your heart scare of most things and
people s
Letting others control you to do things that are not in
your best interest or are harmful to others
Scared of being successful
Doing things for money and not caring who it hurts as
long as you get paid
Making the same mistakes over and over
Realizing you are suffering and in self-denial
Refusing to change what you need to change
In jail or trying to get there fast
Getting your ass beat up by your partner
Being abused and hoping to survive it
Living your life in the past
Doing negative, stupid stuff others want you to do
Thinking the answer is in he bottle or drug

In Conclusion

The list above is long, but opens our minds to things we
sometime do not think about or dismiss as not
consequential. How to change all of that to living well is
to recognize who you are and where you are and to
wake up and change what you need or want to change
for the best. Some choose to suffer, others are forced;
what are you? Love of self requires us to know and try
to live well if we can. It is all up to us. Some do not

know what to do, once you know, you can elect to do or not do, take action or not take action.

Action To No-action

Action no action
Action no action
Learn not what you know
Know what you need to learn
Be ready inaction
Be forward action
Take your time
Benefits are full
Doubt is less
Action more
Dream the way
Each and every day
Rest on your laurels
Stay put in action
Breathe take it easy
Action is allowed
But need to know how to do
If needed
It is you
Not others that need to take action
Procrastinate not inaction
Briefly wade thru the mire
On to the rise up the mountain
As we take action
Knowing we can learn
What we need to know
To take action
From inaction to action

XIII

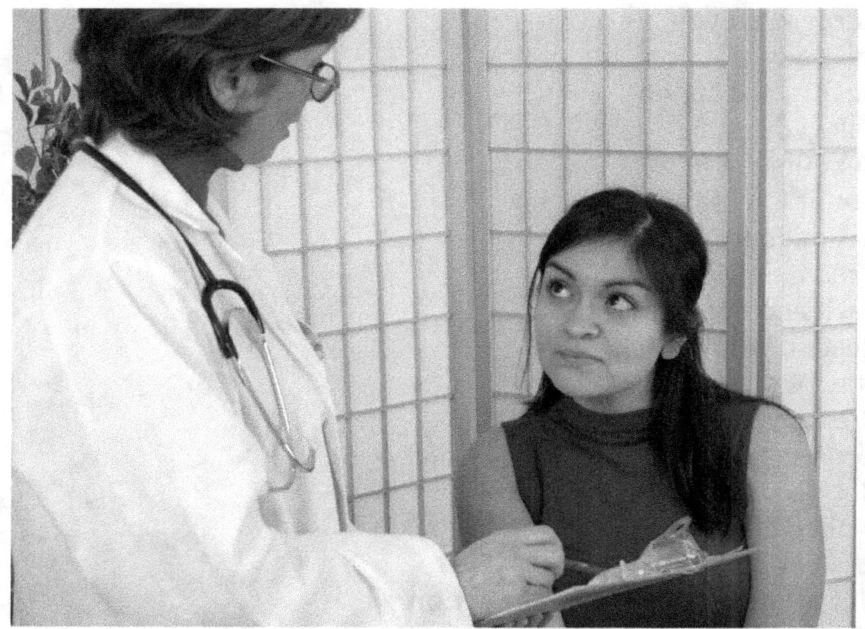

Health Practitioner

Are You Living Well?

In order to live well, one must be able to recognize how they are living now at this moment. Again, we ask, are we healthy? Are we sick? Are we in balance? Do we have things on our minds that are less than healthy? Are these things on our minds making us sick? How do we feel? How do we feel each and every day? Do we get up in the morning with a smile or a frown? Are we thinking thoughts that heal us, or make us unhappy or sick? Are we happy or unhappy? Do we know how to live and live well? What do we need to feel and be healthy? Do you believe you can be healthy, happy and live well? What is in your heart? All of these questions must be acknowledged and answered, even if only to our own selves privately. This is a part of us being aware or awake and not blind or into self-denial. Many people are not aware of their own circumstances for a variety of reasons, or know, but are using their denial ability.

Awareness

What are you aware of concerning your health and life environment? Are you getting regular checkups every year by your local Doctor? In between, are you aware of your health, how you are doing, and if there are issues you are aware of? Have you paid attention to these, or have you ignored them? Have you addressed any health problems or issues? It is ok if we recognize or are aware of health issues and we move to address and remove them. This is our job, to make sure we are healthy, and if not, to address the problems and heal ourselves in order to maintain optimum health. Awareness is the first step. For example, if you are coughing every day and this extends past a few weeks into a few months, it is important for us to try to identify what is causing the problem and correct it, instead of continuing to cough for months and not do anything about it. If you are not sure of the cause of the problem, you can seek advice from a medical professional or alternative health provider. If you go to the toilet once or twice a week, then, instead of assuming that you are ok, you should seek advice or determine what can correct the problem naturally, such as drinking more water or adding fiber to your diet. We are aware of it if we cut our finger, but act like we are not aware if we have a simple cough for months or a pain that is increasing and not going away. Our awareness of our physical condition is very important, and it provides information to our own self that we need to address any situation that appears to be out of balance or out of order. Ignoring it doesn't make it go away. What is more important to ourselves? Going to the party, working 80 hours a week, being rich or our health? It is quite clear it is our health. If we become aware of a problem, we should not panic immediately and rush to get it cut out or think we cannot heal. We should be calm, garner all the information and assistance, and then determine the best course of action to be taken.

Health and Wealth

What is important, money or health? One can have lots of money to buy many toys, but one cannot buy health. Steve Jobs had billions in the bank, but could not buy health. We understand that if you have money, you can buy great medical care, but you cannot buy health. If you have no money, you may not be able to procure great medical services, so it is wise to take care of yourself; if you are poor but healthy, you have wealth. In many countries, people do not have a lot of money to buy premium health care, so they take care of themselves in order to not get sick or require expensive medical services. They recognize that being healthy is important, so they make sure that they stay in balance, stay aware of their general health and, when any problems arise, they address it quickly in order to get back to balance and optimum health. They try to do something every day to maintain optimum health. They are aware that their health is their wealth! They focus on maintaining their health and healing what may ail them on any given day. They do this by using natural and alternative means. This is part of their living well. They then try to maintain that health all the time and not just as a reaction to some temporary incident. They also realize to not worry, live well as they can, and be happy.

Happiness

Why have you not made me happy? I am expecting others to make me happy. When this does not happen, I am sad or depressed; my expectations have been dashed and my faith in the one who is supposed to make me happy has failed. HA! Dream on. No one is supposed to make you happy or sad. You are supposed to make you happy. Waiting or hoping for someone to make you happy is setting yourself up to be disappointed, and then sad or depressed. Many people are walking around depressed because they relied on someone else to do the job you are supposed to do for yourself, but you gave it up, so someone has control over you and your happiness. Then, you blame them instead of blaming yourself, getting over it and taking charge of your own life and will.

The part of living well is you realizing you are in charge of your life, not someone else sitting on your throne controlling you. You need to understand you and who is in charge of you.

List of Live-Well Criteria

Choose to live well by making better or different choices
In good health
Exercise at least 3 to 5 times a week
Rest properly
Relax
Calm
Satisfied with what you have
Being present in the moment
Not focused on the past, such as what I could have or should have done
Not hating
Love in the heart
Putting you first in the equation
Eating properly and enjoying what you eat
Moderation in your eating and drinking choices
Healthy relationships with friends and/or family
Viewing the future with hope and positive optimism
Removing or eliminating negative thinking and/or relationships
Happy home
Balance between work and play

Changing your mind about just letting stuff happen to you, like you have no control
You are happy with your decisions and choices
Not regretting your life or decisions
Being present and not living in the past
Deciding what makes you happy and doing it
Not doing negative, stupid stuff others want you to do

Opportunity

We all have the opportunity to live well, but our criteria of what it means is different for most. Many times it is based on monetary terms. This is a misnomer, because one can live well without being rich or well off. True, one can buy luxuries, but luxuries do not mean you are living well. Living well requires good health, some wisdom, intelligence, understanding, relationships, outlook and an in-look at life and one's circumstances. It also requires what a person's needs and wants are, and how obtainable they are. It is also based on realism, and the reality of the present moment in time and current circumstances. For example, one may feel that they need and want a Lear jet and yacht, but it is not feasible because they have no place to live or any money. In another case, one may want a relationship, but they do not know how to keep a relationship together. One may want good health and to live well, but they ingest harmful drugs every day. One may want to buy a hundred thousand dollar watch, only to then suffer from the stress of worrying about it.

The idea is that we can know realistically what we need, and can control our wants and maintain our health and the health of fruitful relationships. We can also become well rounded and in balance. We can learn what it is to live well and teach ourselves to conduct or change our life to one of balance, good health, and living well, even if we do not have riches to try and buy this and that. We can make decisions to help ourselves be happy. We can be satisfied with what we have and appreciate where we are at the present moment, and then add the changes we need to in order to appreciate our life better and enjoy it more, even without financial riches. For example, taking a date to the park for a walk can be helpful and enjoyable, even though we did not spend any money. Once, a friend of mine was upset because he wanted to take his lady friend out on a date, but had no money, I suggested he take his friend for a walk and enjoy the park, which was free. He took the advice, and his date was a success. We can enjoy each other's company and be happy with ourselves. Happiness comes within, not from outside approval. You can maintain your health by eating well, resting, exercising and enjoying yourself, no matter what you are doing. We can do activities that make us happy, but do not worry our relatives and friends. We can do things and activities that will keep us healthy, safe and in balance. We can make ourselves happy; it is our decision, since happiness comes from within and otherwise cannot be purchased in your local department store.

In Conclusion

Loving ourselves, and our lives, goes a long way toward living well. I start by looking at and loving what I see in the mirror each and every day. I let go of the fear of living and being, and so can you. I focus on the present moment, the present day, not on past stuff! So, how do I do all of this? Get out of the way.

Feel Free and Live Well

Freedom
Free to heal
Free to be
Free to like
Free to be me
Free to see
Who is in front of me?
Free to learn
Free to discern
Free to gain
Knowledge of what it takes
To heal
To feel
Better after I change my behavior
I am sick
I am healed
I have revealed
That I need help
This time I felt
It was of time
To stop
To not cope
To let go
Of what I think about
I release the hate
The grudge
The pain
I am sane
Now that I refrain
From the need to smoke

I can cope
Without the smoke
I am not a dope
I get a chance
To take a glance
At my life
As I change to health
Because health is my wealth
And I am rich
This is an cinch
To understand
My wealth
For myself
Is within my realm
Beneath my feet
Up to the sky
I now can fly
For I have chose
Health
The wealth
For all including myself
If I only believe
And see
As I receive
The information I need
As I strive and dwell on how to live well

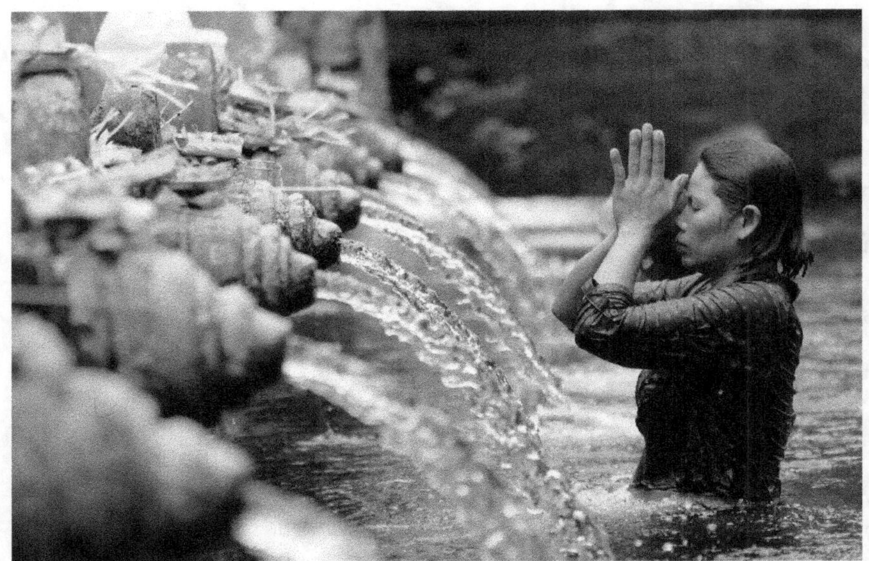

To the Source

Get Out of Your Own Way

Who is in your way? Who is stopping you from living well? No one is in your way. Getting out of your own way is the imperative. Many times, one can change if they want to, but they stop themselves because they are either:

- Stuck on stupid
- Have given up
- No faith in their ability
- Do not believe
- Weak willed
- Scared they may succeed
- Are not goal oriented
- Afraid, scared of change or refuse to change
- Like pain and suffering or drama

- Thinking negative thoughts of I cannot
- Do not know where to begin
- No plan
- Do not think they deserve to live well
- Not motivated

Self-Motivation

The list above covers some reasons why we are not motivated. We can motivate you to begin, challenge yourself, and succeed in changing your mind about what you deserve. You know you deserve to live well. Living well is not about money, it is about health and, balance; that is the real abundance. We know you must also do the basic things to live (such as pay bills), but the most basic is the idea that you deserve to live a healthy and well life by taking good care of you and your family. People have to motivate themselves into doing and being. Nobody can make you live well. It is a conscious decision that you deserve it and to be happy, and you then do those things that can facilitate you living well. They can be complex, or as simple as exercising or walking every day. Or, it can be using your will to stop smoking or to study a trade or get a college degree. Whatever it is, you can use your mind to think the proper thoughts and live well. Making it happen is the self-motivation you need to get it done. If you cannot do it on your own, get some help.

Understanding Why to Live Well

What do you deserve in this life? To suffer, to prosper, to survive, or to live well and love yourself and others? What do you think you deserve: to suffer, or to live abundantly? What you think you deserve is important. Some think they do not deserve anything, while others think they deserve only the best, why does one think differently? It is the value they place on themselves. What value do you place on your self worth? If you think you deserve the best, you are correct. If you think any less, then you need to have a discussion to determine what you really deserve. Living well is the least we deserve, and we should be able to do what it takes to accomplish that; it starts with our health when we are young, and when we are older as an adult or senior citizen. This includes whether we have or do not have money to buy all the luxuries we may desire. Just like you can belong to an expensive health club or you can just exercise outside in the park or at home. Understand you deserve to live well and be happy. Living well is for everyone at any age, young or ancient.

Living Well is Living Longer

Living well does mean living longer. One of the benefits of living well is learning to do the things that will help us to live healthier and to live longer. We cannot control when we come or go, but while we are here, we can live well with the understanding we deserve. As we do the things or activities that will help us to maintain a balanced lifestyle, it improves the quality of our choices that directly and indirectly affect our lifestyle.

Can we all live well? It is possible. Start by thinking correctly that we can, and start to live as well as we can. Some call it aging gracefully, which is a part of living well, and it is for everybody. Doing the correct things, such as eating properly, resting, exercising, and having good relationships, will help. Yes, we need to include friends and family.

Living Well, Living Longer Requirements

We all want to live well longer and want to add to our wellness and abundance, but probably do not reflect on what is required. It is simple, but we must be cognizant of the criteria and make sure we understand our part and do not expect these things to be given to us by someone else. These requirements are "no-excuses" criteria that we can be mindful of and make sure we are adding them to our abundant life. Simple things like resting, drinking water, being calm, not worrying, we all have in our power to enact and accomplish.

Listed below are a few more criteria or properties that those who have lived a long time follow.

Physical Properties
Breathe
Exercise
Stretch
Movement
Rest
Eat nutritious foods
Drink sufficient water

Herbs
Not overdoing partying
Refrain from dangerous drugs, legal or illegal
Don't ingest poisons

Mental and Emotional Properties
Calm
Not worrying
Lessen stress
Use brain
Mindfulness of self and surroundings and environment
Rest your mind
Don't be depressed
Satisfaction with what you have
Lessen greed
Positive relationships
Relax
Don't focus on nonsense outside; wars, politics, injustice
Love yourself
Do not live in the past; be present

In Conclusion

These are things that are supposed to be mindful as we journey through life experiencing the Dao. Don't take the above criteria as a given, not realizing we must make sure we include these properties in our everyday lifestyles. Taking these for granted like the breath we breathe doesn't make them automatic unless we are mindful of what we do, and include on a daily basis. Like making sure we drink water, turn off the TV and get rest, walk, and don't worry about every little thing. Easy to say, but maybe harder to do; yet must be done. So, mull over them and add to them, but be mindful of our daily activities.

Live Well and Prosper

Live well and prosper is not just a fancy saying for those who are rich or are the "haves" versus the "have nots." It is for everyone to abide by and enjoy. You can live well and deserve it. Don't beat yourself or let others tell you that you are not deserving, only them. This is no secret sauce. It is available for all to think about and be mindful of how they are living. I used to ask the question to many, "How are you living?" Then I would say, no matter what answer they gave, "Don't worry, be happy," then go on my way. Just so it would register in their minds to think about the words and apply them to their mindfulness.

You Be Mindful of These

Respect yourself
Use your willpower
Moderation is the key
Eat naturally and nutritiously
Breathe deeply
Exercise everyday if possible or at least 4 time a week
Rest and get your sleep
Cleanliness is vital
Do no harm to self and others

Nature helps, near the sea, in the forest and on the mountain
Control your emotions
Think positive thoughts and dismiss negative thoughts
Let go of past stuff
Meditate
Take care of your body
Do not worry, or hurry; be happy
Love yourself
Enjoy your life
See the good
Appreciate what you have
Be loving to yourself and others

Go over the ideas listed above and just contemplate them as you go about your day. Are you doing these already, or do you need to incorporate some of these into your daily routine?

In Conclusion

People say "be well" and should also say "live well" to each other as a reminder of our goal in life. Remember, "live well" is an attitude based on knowing you deserve it. As a gift, give it to yourself and your family. Believe, trust, faith, test yourself; yes, you can. Start today!

How to Start Today

Do not think you cannot do. You can live well. Yes, you can start right now by instituting some of these ideas, and activities today. Let's not wait or procrastinate, let's start with these suggestions:

Start a (new) hobby
Watch less TV
Listen to music
Read a book
Get more sleep
Take more walks
Get out into nature
Travel more visit other places around the world
Eat more nutritious and organic foods
Eat slowly
Stretch your body
Take better care of your teeth
Get a massage
Laugh more
Be happy with you
Think positive
Develop good relationships
Make goals and write them down
Then act upon the goals
Quit smoking
Do not let social media control you and your thoughts
Say yes I can
Don't Worry Be Happy!

In Conclusion

What Helps You to Live Well (condensed)

Exercise

Exercise keeps the body supple, flexible, and maintains excellent circulation, which includes the health and strength of the muscles and the tendons.

Rest and sleep
Proper rest and sleep helps us to rest the body and to improve our energy

Water
Water is the elixir of life, for all living things need water for nourishment, for cleansing and growth

Food and Herbs
Foods and herbs help to nourish our bodies for optimum health and healing our bodies to keep our organs strong

Love and Inner Peace
Love keeps the heart happy as we appreciate our life, relationships and nature as it celebrates us everyday. Love yourself

Stop Worrying: Be happy
Our minds need to be free from strife and the stress of stuff we deal with on a daily basis that causes us to forget to live well and just be happy we are alive

Being Present
It is the being in the present moment that counts; and we must try to make the most of it, and do not focus on the stuff that has passed in the past.

What to Do For Tomorrow?

Drink water
Drink Gatorade
Drink wine
It is all fine
Salt of the earth
Sugar so sweet
What is good or bad for me?

Waste not want not
Need this take that
Under the amount overdose
Need more or less
What is good, bad or the best?

Is it medicine, is it surgery
Is it ok or is it an emergency
I know that I can
I know not what I need to know
I am ok I think
I wonder if I am
What do you think?

Is it real?
Is it fake?
Is the pain real?
Is it a mistake?
What do you think?
Oh it is not you
It is your pain not mine

I am the doctor
You are the patient
Or you unaware
Is all in a haze
Are you patient

Or are you in a hurry

Save me save the children
From inoculations
That creates a need
To now heal
When I was already well
Enough to see
That drug is not for me

Don't make excuses
Take action
What to do
Use commonsense
Or the old wife's tale
And a little butter
Garlic and honey
That is sweet
And it heals too
I am happy
No side effect then

I can go about my day
My health in tact
Are (feeling) better
Or worse
Don't you know?
Need someone else to tell you

Wake up, you are in charge
Of who, you fool
Not me, I am just the advisor
You are on the throne
Or don't you know you are in charge
Of you and your wealth

Can't take it away from you
Because it is your health

The real wealth
Lead and follow
Save it for another day
So you will have it for tomorrow tomorrows.

The Metaphor: Using the Idea of "Live Well"

Using the idea of living well as a metaphor and an outcry to all to choose to improve their health and begin to decrease the effects of non-communicable dis-eases (NCDs). NCDs can be decreased by instituting effective programs for all, whether they are rich or poor, or with health or no health insurance. The idea that people can prevent most health related dis-eases is paramount. We need to not rely solely on scientific medicine; we can do better by instituting preventative programs that promote healing, exercises, and education projects and are inclusive, that will move people and communities to help each other to do what it takes to live healthier lives and live well.

We must begin to teach and educate and train others to develop the practice of living well. Part of this leads us to the "Healing Project: How to be Healthy and Live Well."

"Bacon, soda & too few nuts tied to big portion of US deaths

AP

Lindsey Tanner, AP Medical Writer 7 hours ago

mega share CommentsSign in to like Reblog on TumblrShareTweetEmail

CHICAGO (AP) -- Gorging on bacon, skimping on nuts? These are among food habits that new research links with deaths from heart disease, strokes and diabetes.

Overeating or not eating enough of the 10 foods and nutrients contributes to nearly half of U.S. deaths from these causes, the study suggests.

"Good" foods that were under-eaten include: nuts and seeds, seafood rich in omega-3 fats including salmon and sardines; fruits and vegetables; and whole grains.

"Bad" foods or nutrients that were over-eaten include salt and salty foods; processed meats including bacon, bologna and hot dogs; red meat including steaks and hamburgers; and sugary drinks.

The research is based on U.S. government data showing there were about 700,000 deaths in 2012 from heart disease, strokes and diabetes and on an analysis of national health surveys that asked participants about their eating habits. Most didn't eat the recommended amounts of the foods studied.

The 10 ingredients combined contributed to about 45 percent of those deaths, according to the study.

It may sound like a familiar attack on the typical American diet, and the research echoes previous studies on the benefits of heart-healthy eating. But the study goes into more detail on specific foods and their risks or benefits, said lead author Renata Micha, a public health researcher and nutritionist at Tufts University.

The results were published Tuesday in the Journal of the American Medical Association.

Micha said the foods and nutrients were singled out because of research linking them with the causes of death studied. For example, studies have shown that excess salt can increase blood pressure, putting stress on arteries and the heart. Nuts contain healthy fats that can improve cholesterol levels, while bacon and other processed meats contain saturated fats that can raise levels of unhealthy LDL cholesterol.

In the study, too much salt was the biggest problem, linked with nearly 10 percent of the deaths. Overeating processed meats and under eating nuts and seeds and seafood each were linked with about 8 percent of the deaths.

The Food and Drug Administration's recent voluntary sodium reduction guidelines for makers of processed foods and taxes that some U.S. cities have imposed on sugar-sweetened beverages are steps in the right direction, Micha said.

A journal editorial said public health policies targeting unhealthy eating could potentially help prevent some deaths, while noting that the study isn't solid proof that "suboptimal" diets were deadly.

The study's recommended amounts, based on U.S. government guidelines, nutrition experts' advice, and amounts found to be beneficial or harmful in previous research.

"Good" ingredients

—Fruits: 3 average-sized fruits daily

—Vegetables: 2 cups cooked or 4 cups raw vegetables daily

—Nuts/seeds: 5 1-ounce servings per week — about 20 nuts per serving

—Whole grains: 2 ½ daily servings

—Polyunsaturated fats, found in many vegetable oils: 11 percent of daily calories

—Seafood: about 8 ounces weekly

"Bad" ingredients

—Red meat: 1 serving weekly — 1 medium steak or the equivalent

—Processed meat: None recommended

—Sugary drinks: None recommended

—Salt: 2,000 milligrams daily — just under a teaspoon.

—

Online:
Diet guidelines: http://tinyurl.com/j5lcrv8

—

Follow AP Medical Writer Lindsey Tanner at
http://www.twitter.com/LindseyTanner
Her work can be found at
http://bigstory.ap.org/content/lindsey-tanner"

XIV

The Healing Project: How to Be Healthy and Live Well Project: achieving optimum health and living well

I Alternative methodologies explored and explained
Herbal/homeopathic remedies prescription
Diet and Nutrition program
Ayurveda and TCM (five element) Balance program
Exercises presented and discussed such as Dao yin and Taijiquan
Recommended or prescribed reading program
Setting individual schedule/programs

II Programmatic Evaluation Results
1.   One month
2.   Three months
3.   Six months
4.   One year

III Understanding Spiritual Health and Why it is Important

IV Your Individual Needs Evaluation

V Discussion Topics Covered: Series

Various topics will be covered and will be determined in the near future.
This is a living project and we will add to it, tweak it and change whatever needs to be changed.

The Dao

The Healing Project
How to Be Healthy and Live Well

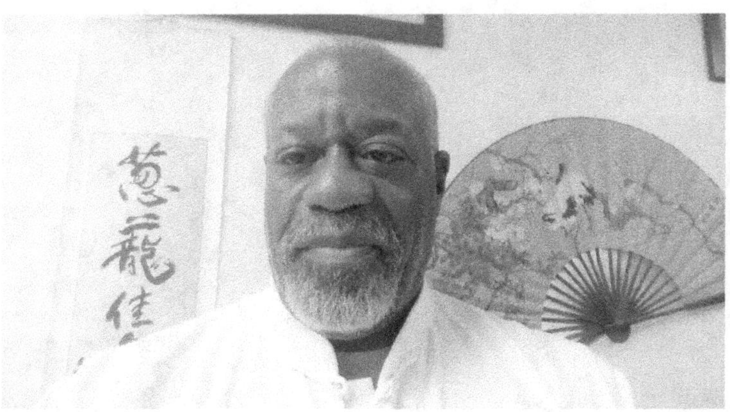

About the Author

Dr. George writes to assist with the spreading of knowledge and light to all who seek to educate themselves on a variety of levels. His previous book on Tortoise: The Way of Longevity is vital for all those who seek to learn more about longevity and insight on what one may do to increase their own longevity. His new book, "the Healing Project: How to be healthy and Live Well" focuses on the basis ideal that we all need to be healthy and to live well. Dr. George is a practitioner and teacher of Chinese internal martial arts. Dr. George Samuels, M.D. (A.M.) is an enlightened and realized Spiritual Master, Guide, Teacher, Healer, Spiritual Coach, Author and Poet, and he is here to teach and help heal those who seek answers and want to learn in order to help others. Dr. George has been providing light, spiritual wisdom, healing, coaching, and spiritual guidance for thousands of people throughout the USA and other countries for more than 30 years. He continues to and is currently helping and healing all who contact him and are seeking Light on the Path. Dr. George provides Insight, Readings, Spiritual Counseling, Coaching and Training Classes, on every level in-person or long distance and includes Qigong Healing, Tai Chi Gong and Internal Boxing.
My Websites:

www.spirituallifesource.com
www.gsamuelsbooksandart.com